Inguinal Hernias and Hydroceles in Infants and Children

Single Surgical Procedures 3

A Colour Atlas of

Inguinal Hernias and Hydroceles in Infants and Children

Caroline M. Doig

W DE G

Walter de Gruyter · Berlin · New York 1984

Caroline M. Doig Ch. M, FRCSE, FRCS; Senior Lecturer in Paediatric Surgery, University of Manchester and Booth Hall Children's Hospital Manchester

Original Publishers: Wolfe Medical Publications Ltd., · London
Exclusive co-publishers for the Federal Republic of Germany and Austria: Walter de Gruyter & Co., Genthiner Strasse 13, D-1000 Berlin 30. 1984.

Printed by Royal Smeets Offset b.v., Weert, Netherlands

Cover design: Rudolf Hübler

General Editor, Wolfe Surgical Atlases:
William F. Walker, DSc, ChM, FRCS (Eng.), FRCS (Edin.), FRS (Edin.)

CIP-Kurztitelaufnahme der Deutschen Bibliothek

Doig, Caroline M.:
A colour atlas of inguinal hernias and hydroceles in infants and children / Caroline M. Doig. –
Berlin; New York: de Gruyter, 1984.
(Single surgical procedures; 3)
ISBN 3-11-010011-8
ISBN 3-11-010010-X (Subskr.-Pr.)
NE: GT

Contents

To my Mother for her constant support and encouragement.

Acknowledgements

I am indebted to my numerous teachers in Paediatric Surgery who taught me the management of baby hernias and hydroceles.

My grateful thanks to my photographer who patiently took numerous photographs of inguinal herniotomies and hydrocele operations, and to my secretary for typing the manuscript.

I wish to acknowledge the help of the Manchester North District Area Health Authority for allowing the use of slides of children admitted to Booth Hall Children's Hospital, Manchester.

Introduction

The operations described in this book are those commonly performed by most paediatric surgeons and those general surgeons, who have a wide experience in dealing with hernias and hydroceles in children.

No surgery should be undertaken in children, let alone babies, without the surgeon having had adequate surgical training. The importance of the team in looking after these children cannot be over emphasised – this includes the anaesthetist, ward and theatre nurses, and surgeons.

Inguinal hernias in children are congenital in nature and therefore are almost always indirect. The hernial sac passes through the deep inguinal ring, the inguinal canal and the superficial ring within the coverings of the cord. By virtue of the anatomy in the baby and infant, the deep and superficial rings are almost superimposed with very little potential inguinal canal. Because of this it is possible to deal with the hernial sac through both inguinal rings without opening the inguinal canal.

Such hernias are more likely to become irreducible, because it is easy for bowel to enter the sac, leading to eventual strangulation. In view of this, hernias in babies and infants under two years of age should always be operated on urgently. In my practice, they undergo surgery on the first available operating list.

Types of inguinal hernia

1

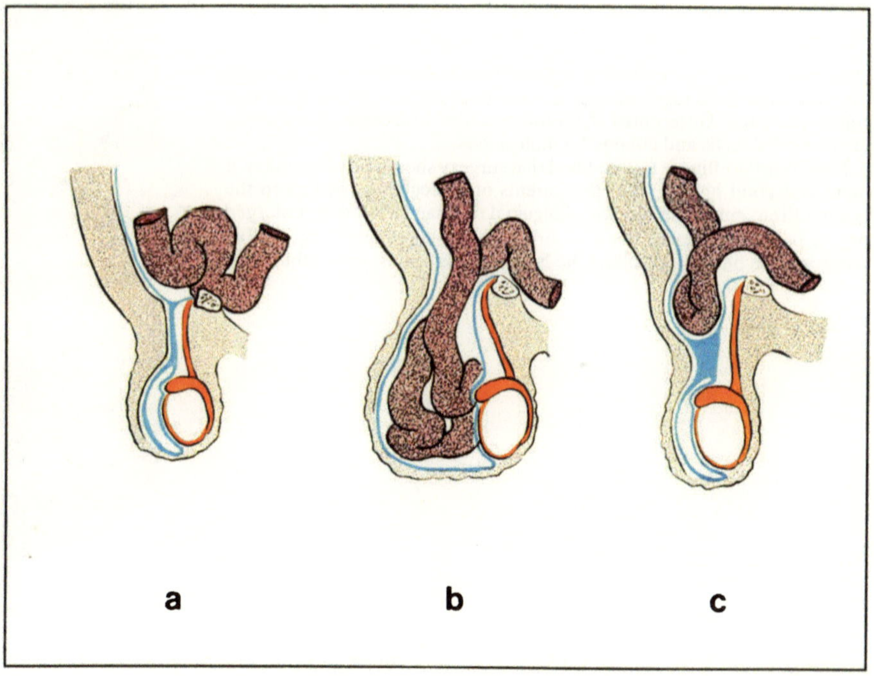

1 Types of inguinal hernia in infants and children.
a) Normal anatomy
b) Complete scrotal indirect hernia
c) Incomplete indirect inguinal hernia

The incidence is 1:50 in boys and 1:400 in girls. Baby hernias occur on the right side in 60 per cent of cases and in 25 per cent on the left side. Because only 15 per cent occur bilaterally, routine bilateral exploration is not carried out unless there is a history of swelling or a wide inguinal ring is felt on the contralateral side.

Diagnosis

Diagnosis is easy in a reducible inguinal hernia, because it is a swelling over the superficial inguinal ring and in the scrotum which reduces with gentle pressure. Differential diagnosis includes hydrocele of the cord, undescended testis and enlarged lymph glands.

Even if no swelling is found, I feel that surgery should be undertaken if there is a good history from the parents of a recurring swelling in the groin. Often, either the superficial inguinal ring can be felt to be enlarged or, on palpating the cord and coverings at the superficial ring, a silky sensation can be felt i.e. rolling the hernial walls against each other.

2

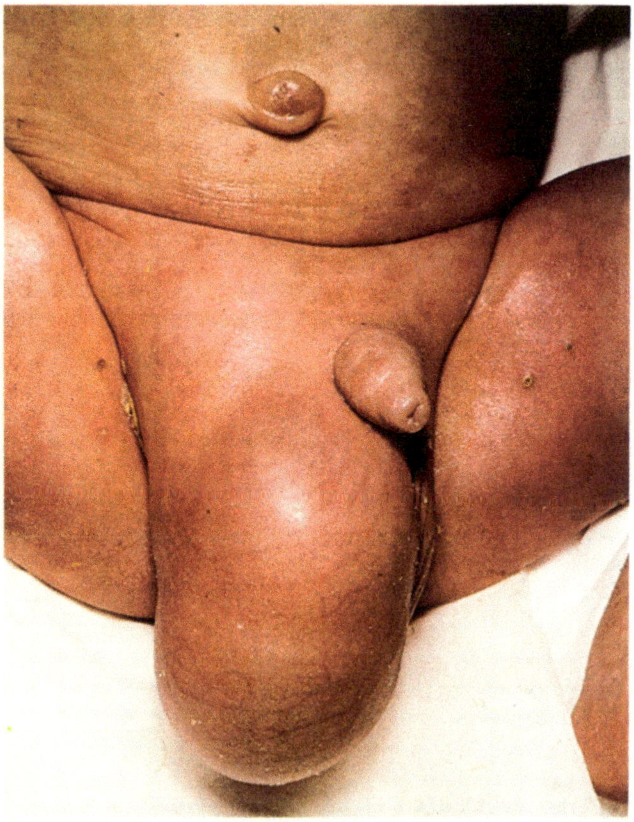

2 Large scrotal inguinal hernia. Such a hernia is easily reducible into the superficial inguinal ring.

3 Bilateral, incomplete inguinal hernias with elevation of testes out of the scrotum.

3

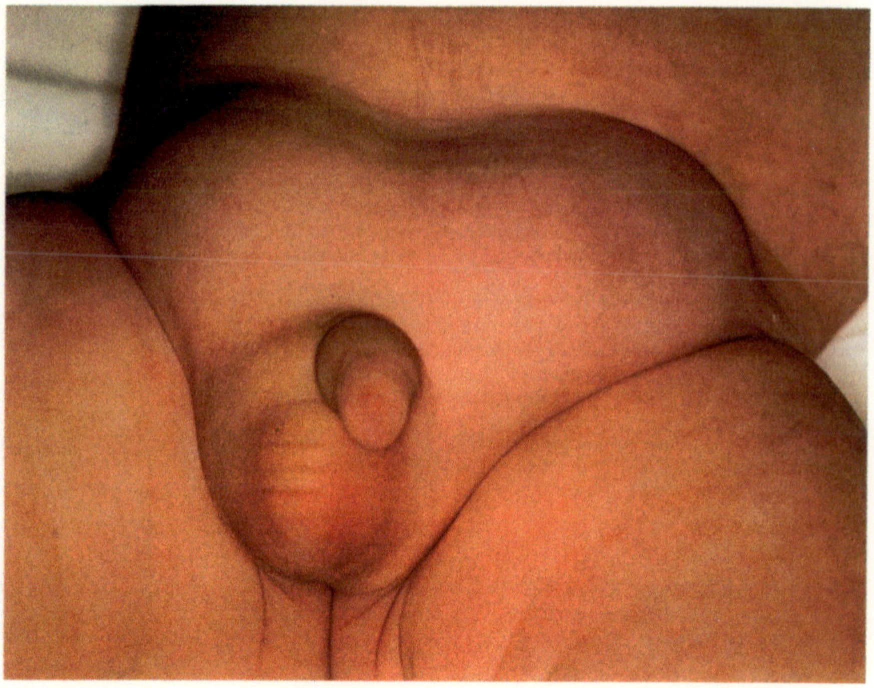

The commonest complication of baby inguinal hernias is incarceration of bowel leading to obstruction, reduction in blood supply and ischaemic bowel. This occurs especially in the very young and premature baby. If missed it leads to perforation, peritonitis, septicaemia and death. Compression of testicular vessels leading to ischaemia and gangrene of the testes can also occur very quickly. The differential diagnosis in such cases include lymphadenitis, acute hydrocele and torsion of testes.

Treatment

Because of the risk of incarceration, baby hernias should be dealt with as soon as they are diagnosed. They should not be put on a waiting-list, but need surgery as a semi-emergency on the next available list. In the older child the risk of damage to bowel or testis is less acute and surgery can be carried out in an elective manner.

Sedation of the child with elevation of the foot end of the bed is usually all that is necessary to allow the more difficult baby hernias to reduce. Gentle traction may also be used. When hernias are reduced by conservative measures, we keep the child in hospital for two to four days to allow oedema to settle, and then perform elective herniotomy before discharging the patient.

The risk of conservative management of incarcerated bowel in a hernial sac is that the necrotic bowel may be returned to the peritoneal cavity following the manual reduction of the hernia. Such children, who are treated conservatively, must be observed closely for the next 6 to 12 hours and may require surgery if it becomes incarcerated again or if physical signs suggest peritonitis.

However, if the hernia does not reduce easily, emergency surgery must follow because of the risk to both the bowel within the hernial sac and the blood supply to the testis.

4

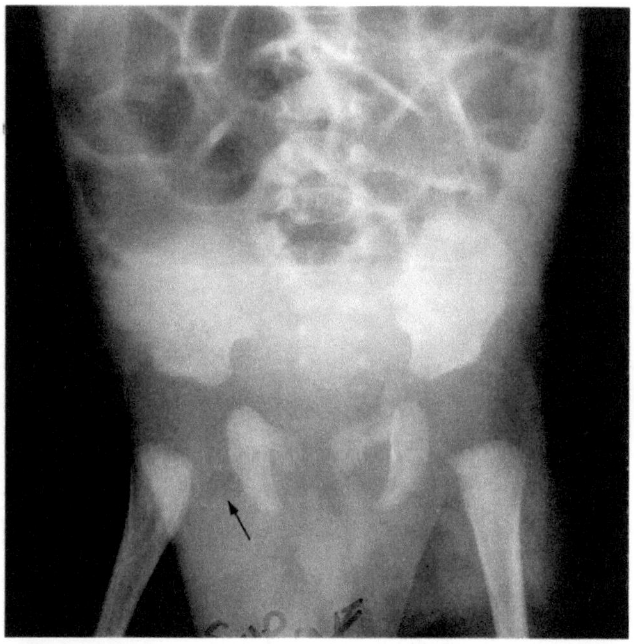

4 Gas bubble in scrotum. Xray of a gas bubble (arrowed) in the scrotum indicative of bowel in the scrotum, which suggests an irreducible hernia. Urgent surgery is a must.

Operation of elective inguinal herniotomy

The following operation can be performed for elective repair of inguinal hernias in all babies and children up to their early teens. It may be necessary in the older child to open the inguinal canal to allow the hernial sac to be completely dissected – the operation becoming similar to that performed in adults.

In the case of elective surgery, the children are admitted as day cases, or at the most for an overnight stay. All children are operated upon under general anaesthesia. No premedication is given to children under one year. Trimeprazine tartrate is used in the older infant and child. All children are intubated and monitored, either on assisted ventilation or spontaneous ventilation with a paediatric circuit. Postoperatively, intramuscular pethidine is given.

5

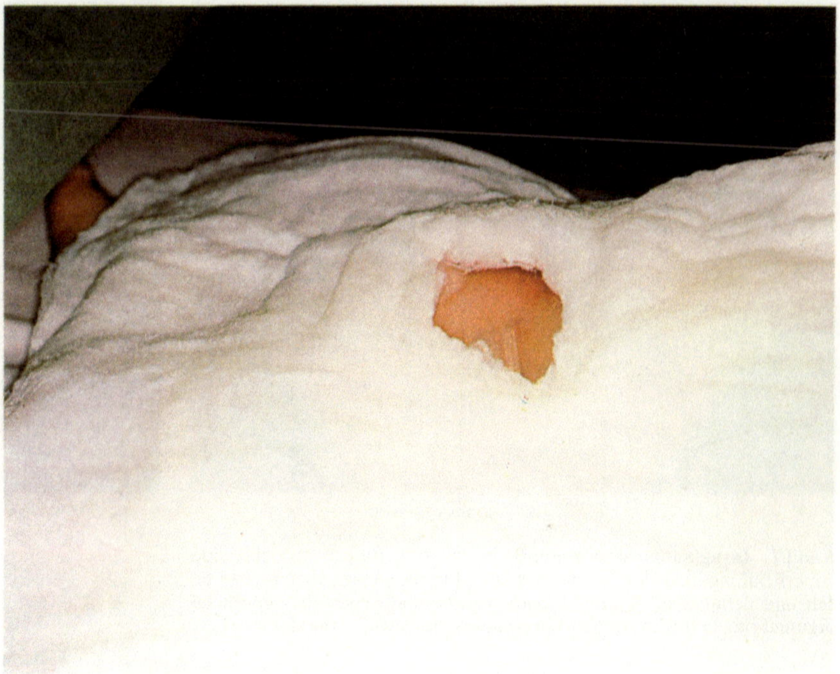

5 **Prevention of hypothermia.** In the baby, especially aged under three months, there is a risk of hypothermia during surgery. These children should be placed on an electric or hot-water blanket. During surgery they are covered with warm, sterile gamgee, under the sterile drapes. A hole is cut to allow the operation to be carried out. With the older child four gamgee pads can be used, leaving the operative field clear.

6

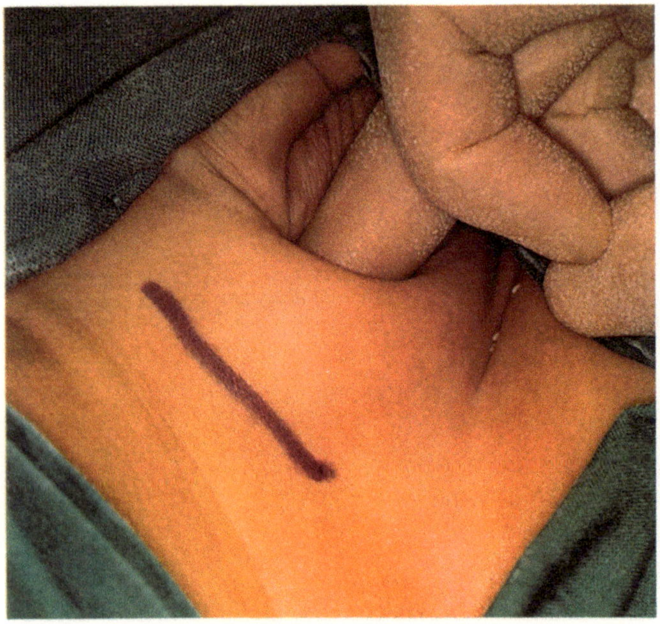

7

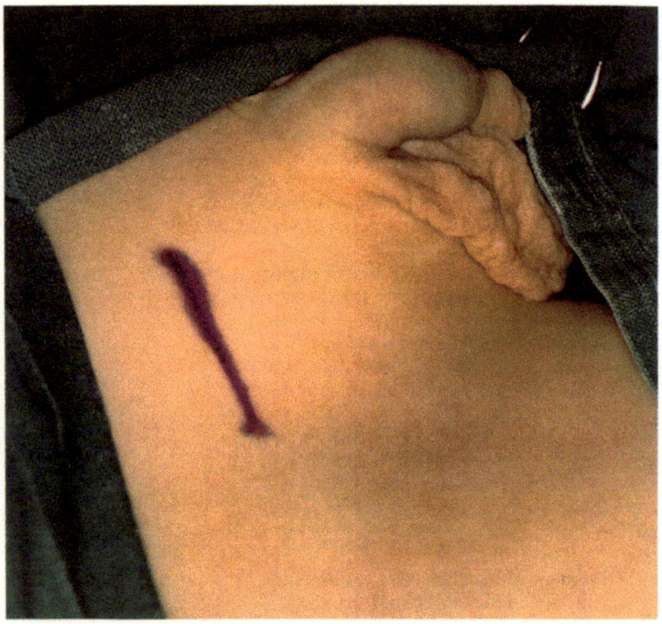

6 and 7 Invagination of scrotum. By invaginating the scrotum, the wide superficial inguinal ring, above and lateral to the pubic tubercle, can be felt and delineated. A short incision can be made over the superficial inguinal ring in the line of the skin crease as indicated by the skin marker.

8

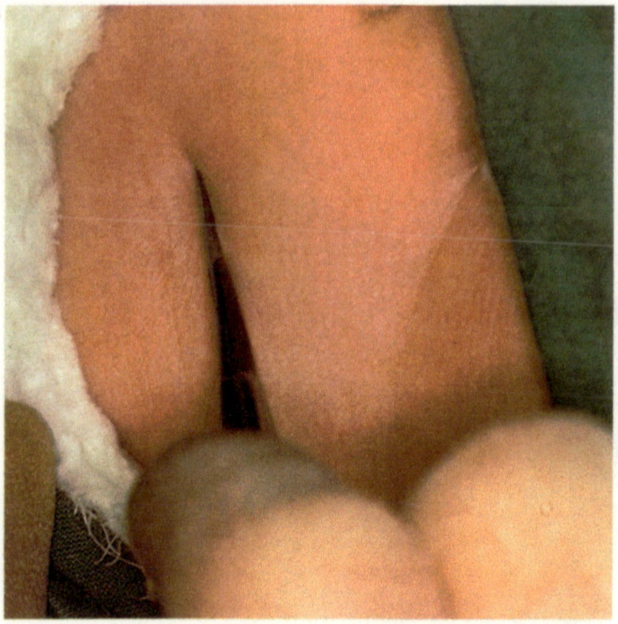

8 In a female child the incision is made over the superficial inguinal ring. If the incision is correctly positioned, neither the superficial epigastric artery nor the ilio-inguinal nerve can be damaged.

9

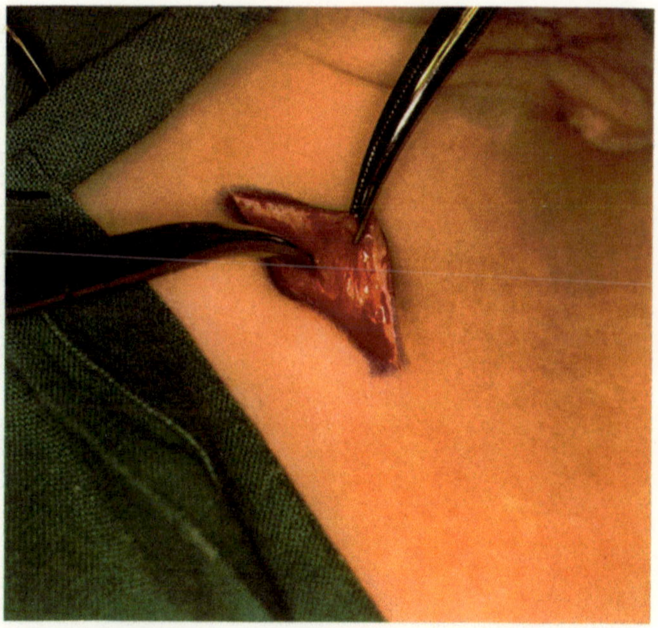

9 Two mosquito clips are placed on either side of the incision on subcutaneous tissues. There is rarely any bleeding. If bleeding does occur, a clip is left for a few minutes and twisted off so as to prevent any need for diathermy. Ligation of vessels is not normally necessary.

10

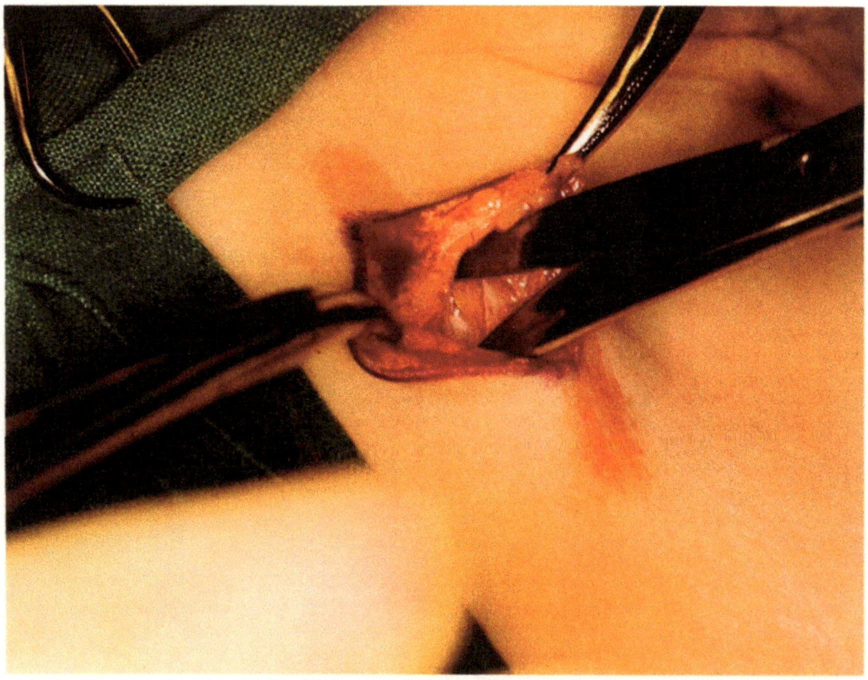

10 The clips are held up by the assistant and blunt dissection, using McIndoe scissors, carried down through the deep fascia towards the superficial inguinal ring.

11

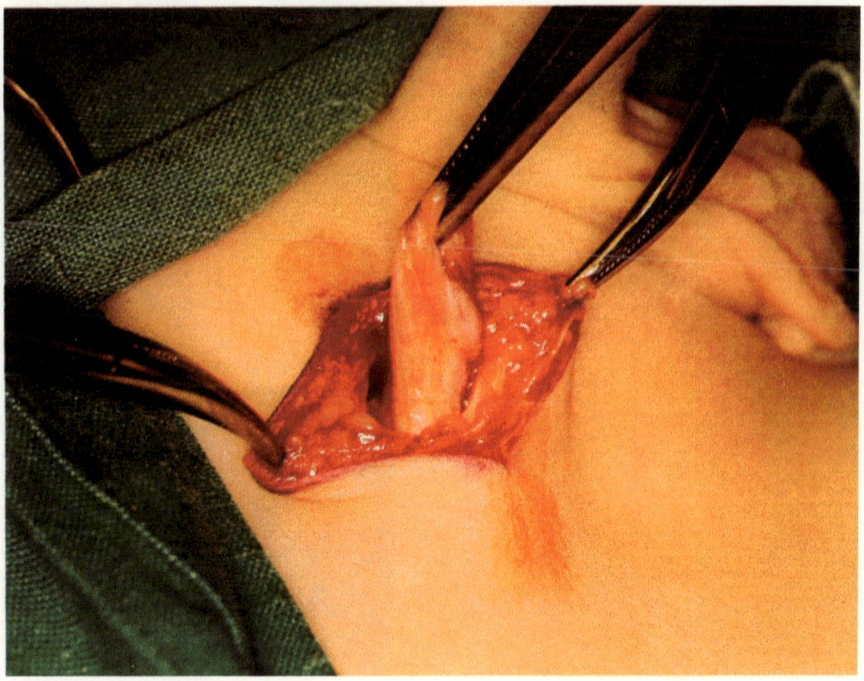

11 After the deep fascia has been opened the superficial ring can be palpated. Blunt dissecting forceps are used to bring out the cord and coverings through the wound. This is possible, even if the child is fat, because there is only the spermatic cord with its coverings coming through the superficial inguinal ring. In a girl, only fat and the hernial sac appear at the ring.

12

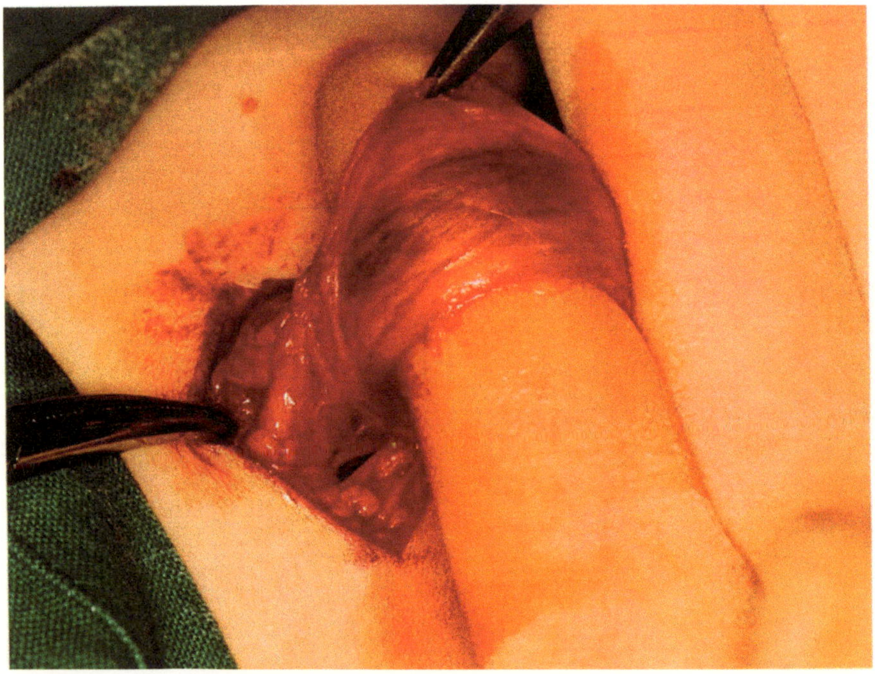

12 By blunt dissection, the cord with associated hernia, is freed of surrounding fat, so that it is possible to pass the index finger of the operator through the tissue to allow these structures to lie on top of the index finger.

13

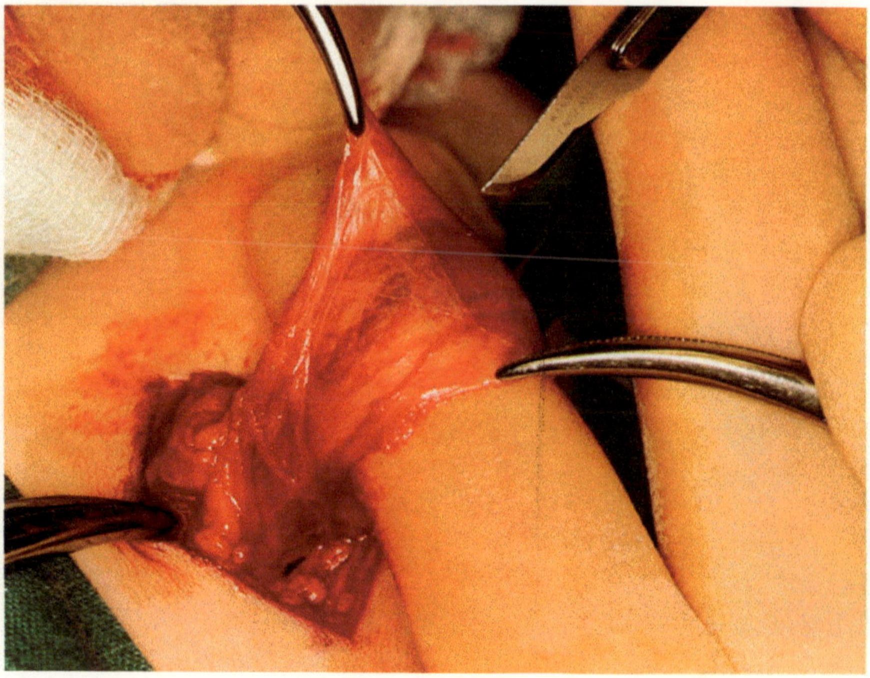

13 Two clips are placed on the coverings i.e. the external spermatic fascia and cremasteric muscle. The clips are held up to put the tissue on tension.

14

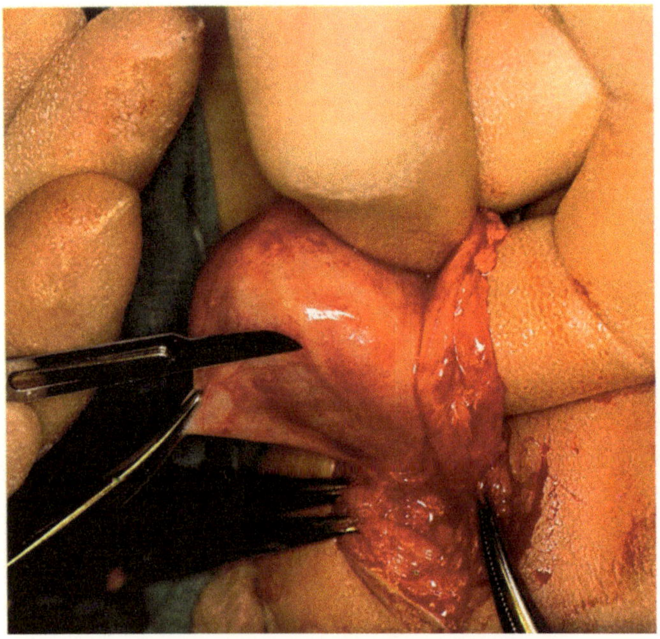

15

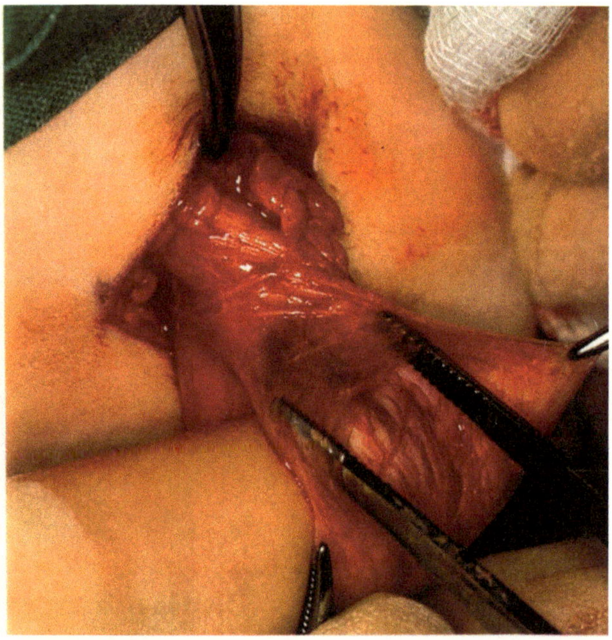

14 This allows the vas to be visualised. Division of these coverings with a knife can then be carried out safely without damage to the vas or testicular vessels. Here the knife is pointing to the vas deferens.

15 Dissection is then carried out proximally to the superficial inguinal ring. The fascia and muscle are lifted up by forceps to allow them to be cut and to give a clear view of the inguinal ring.

16

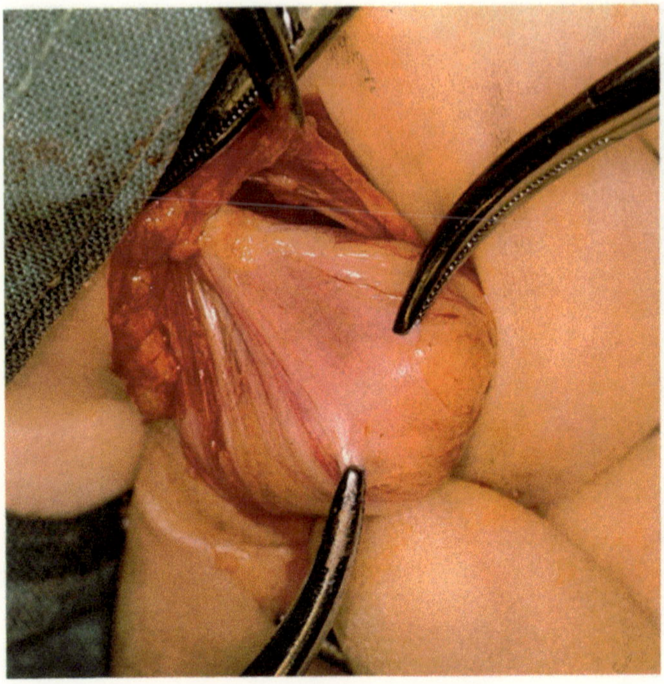

17

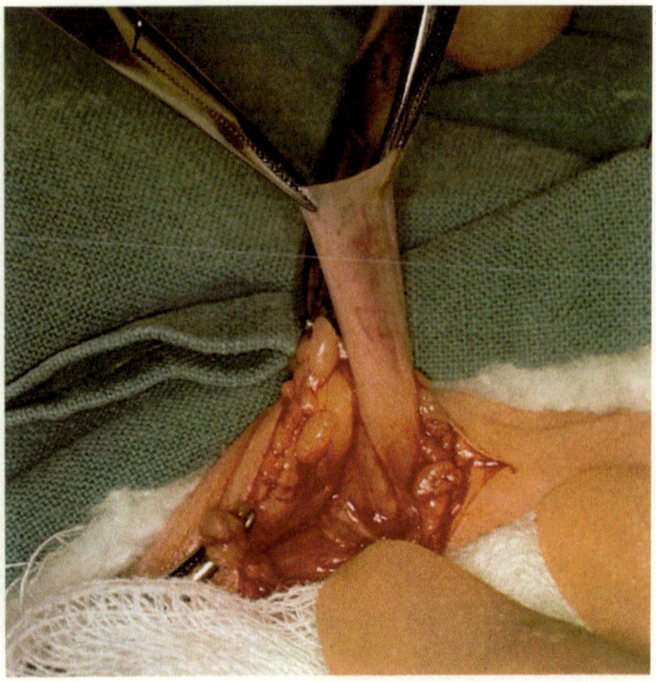

16 In the case of an incomplete hernial sac the outline of the sac can be seen and picked up by mosquito clips.

17 By putting traction on the sac, blunt dissection can be carried out easily using either a dry swab or blunt broad forceps. Care should be taken during this manoeuvre not to damage the vas deferens and the vessels.

18

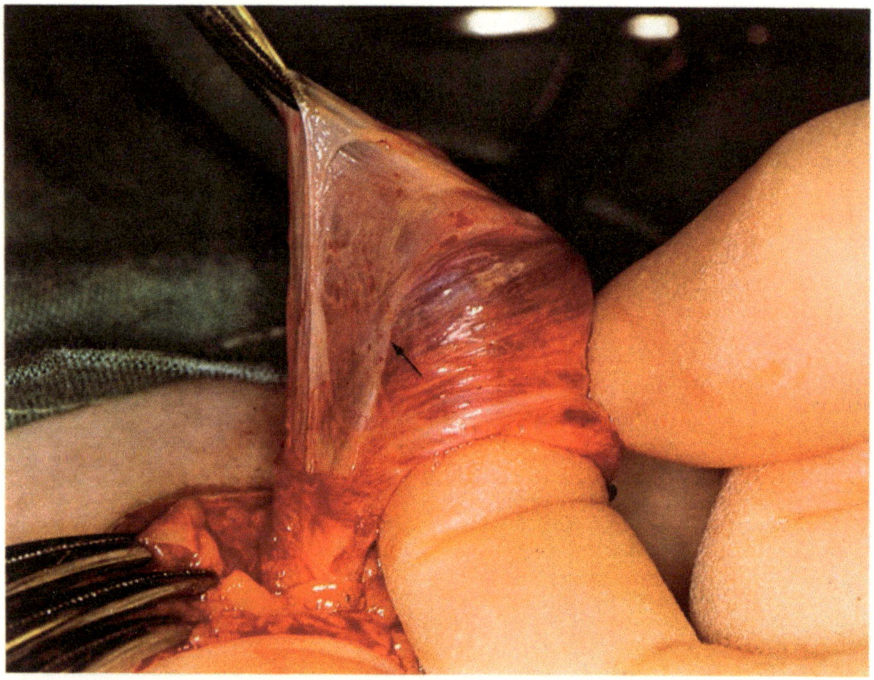

18 Even if the hernia is of the more common scrotal type, the sac can be visualised (arrowed) and separated from the vas and vessels which are lying posterolateral. If care is taken with the very fine sac, it is possible to dissect it free without damage.

19

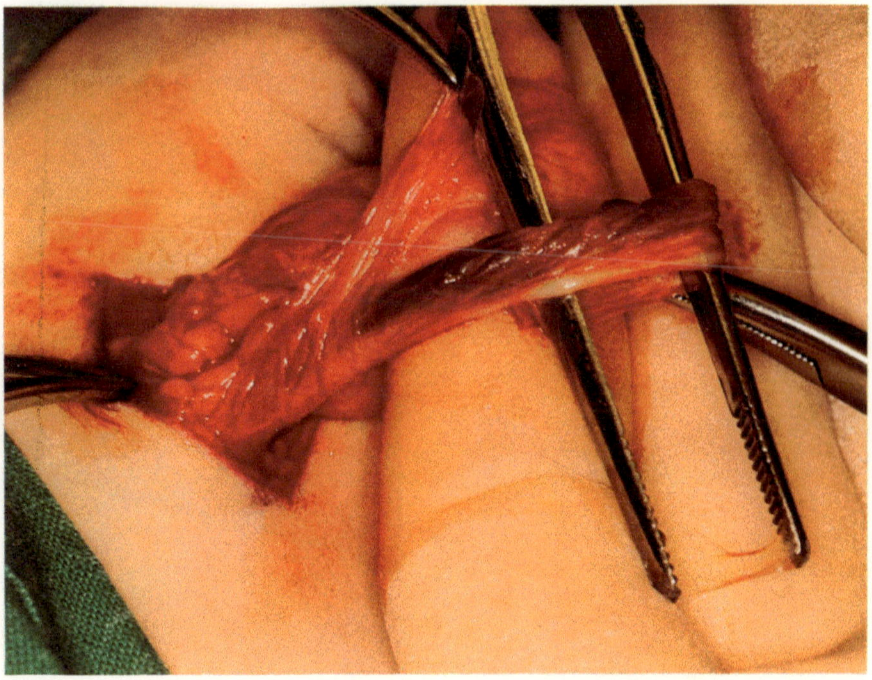

19 Once free, damage to testicular vessels and the vas deferens can be prevented by use of an Allis forceps to keep them clear of the dissection.

20

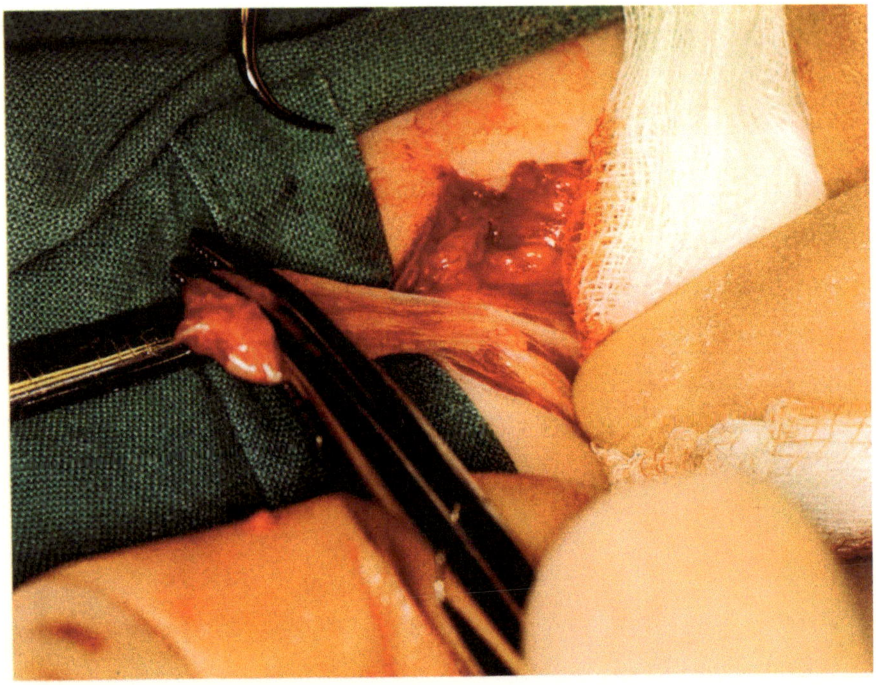

20 Two clips are put on the hernial sac which is then divided distally. Careful dissection downwards towards the inguinal ring can then be carried out as before with a dry swab and the sac on tension.

21

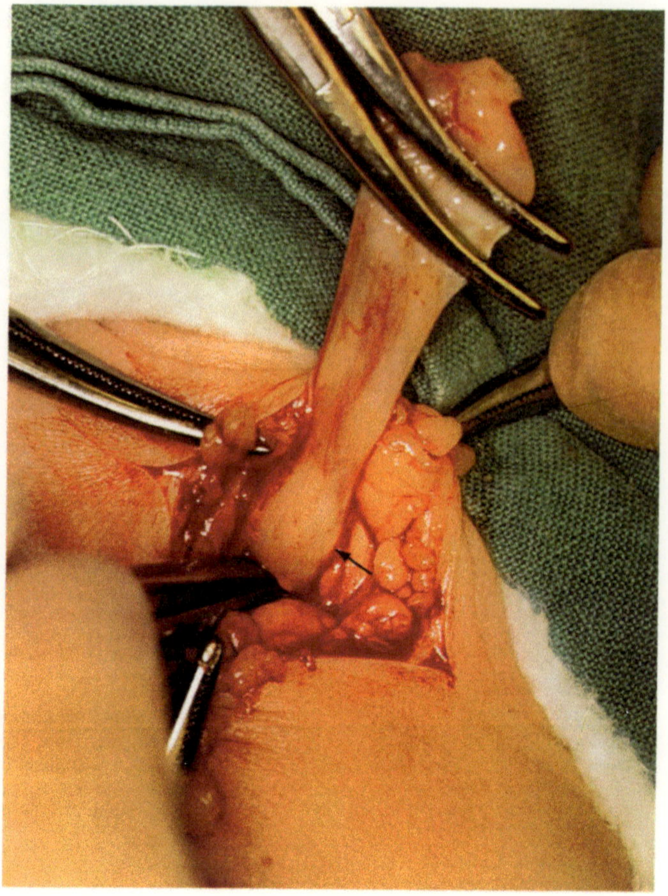

21 If adequate dissection is carried out, a pad of extra-peritoneal fat (arrowed) indicates that the deep inguinal ring has been reached.

22

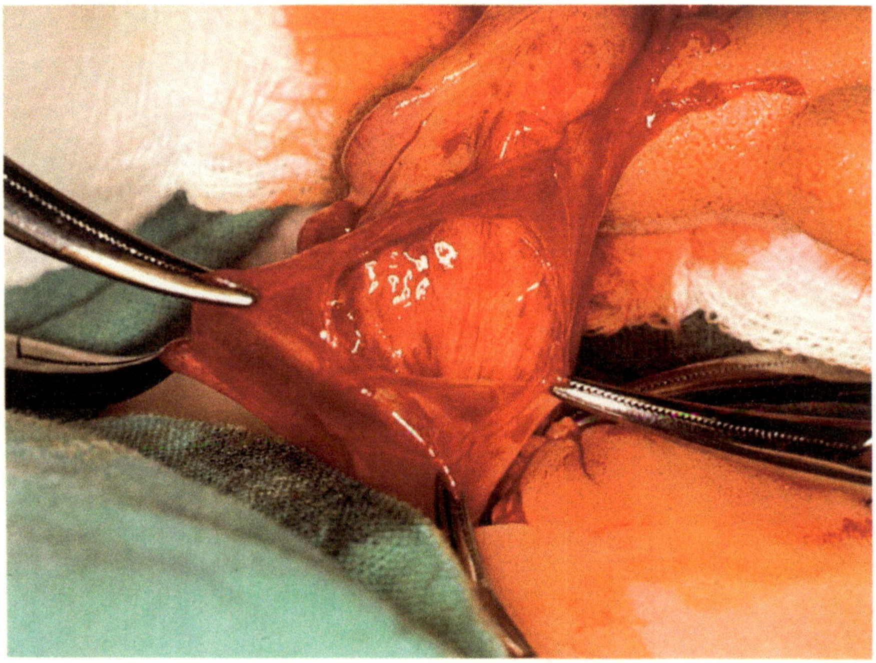

22 Hernial sac damage. However, the hernial sac can be damaged easily during dissection, especially in the case of a very fine sac which can be difficult to visualise. In that case clips may be put on at right angles to the line of the sac to prevent the sac from tearing further towards the peritoneum.

23

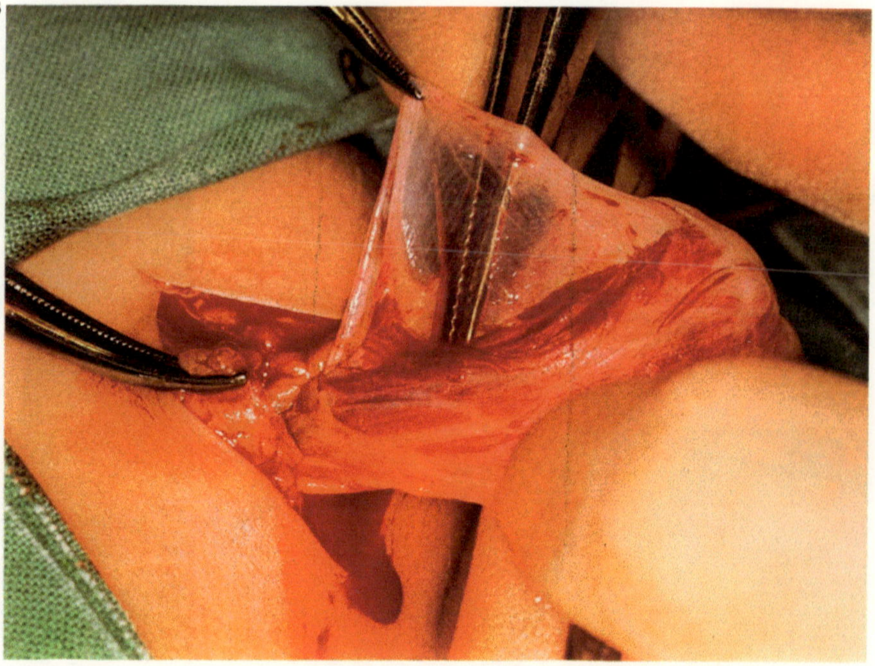

23 If this happens the very fine sac can be dissected bit by bit, clearing it away from the vas and vessels with care, so as not to damage them.

24 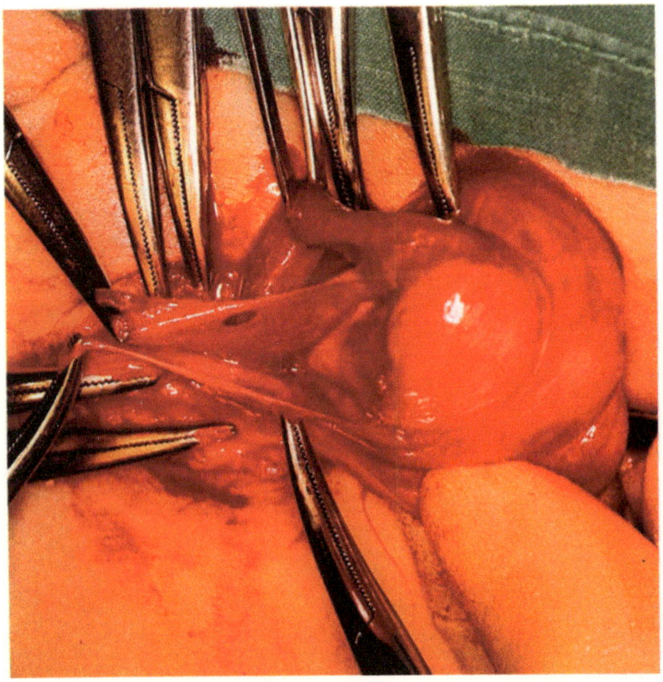

25 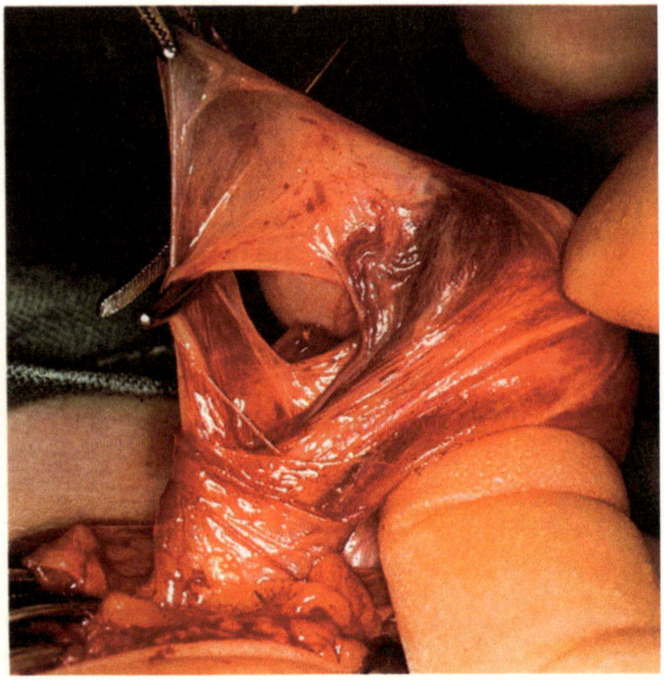

24 By careful dissection, eventually the complete 'ring' of the sac can be seen, lying free from the vessels. In some very small children with 'tissue paper'-like sacs, this may be time consuming.

25 Two clips are placed across the hernial sac which is then divided distally. Dissection is then carried out as before towards the superficial inguinal ring.

26

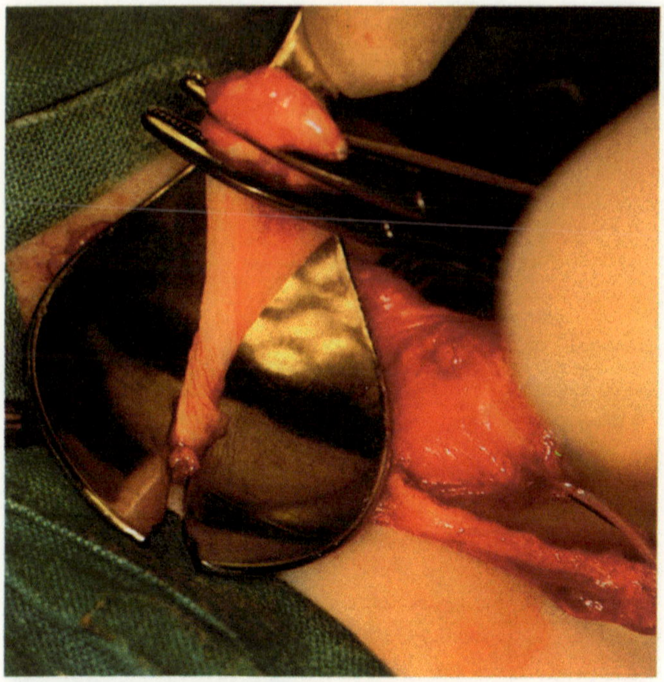

27

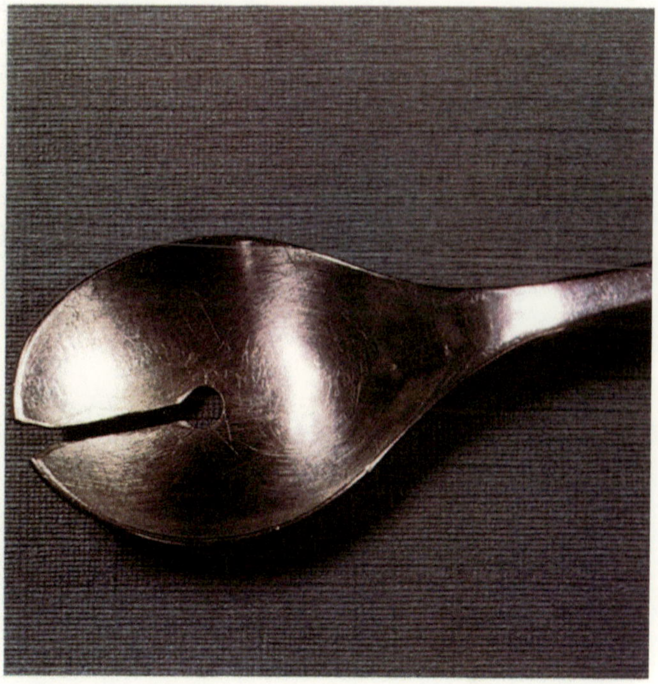

26 The sac whether opened or closed is twisted to return any contents to the peritoneal cavity. A Denis Browne spoon is used to keep the vas and vessels separate from the hernial sac.

27 A Denis Browne spoon. This is an ordinary teaspoon with a groove cut into it.

28

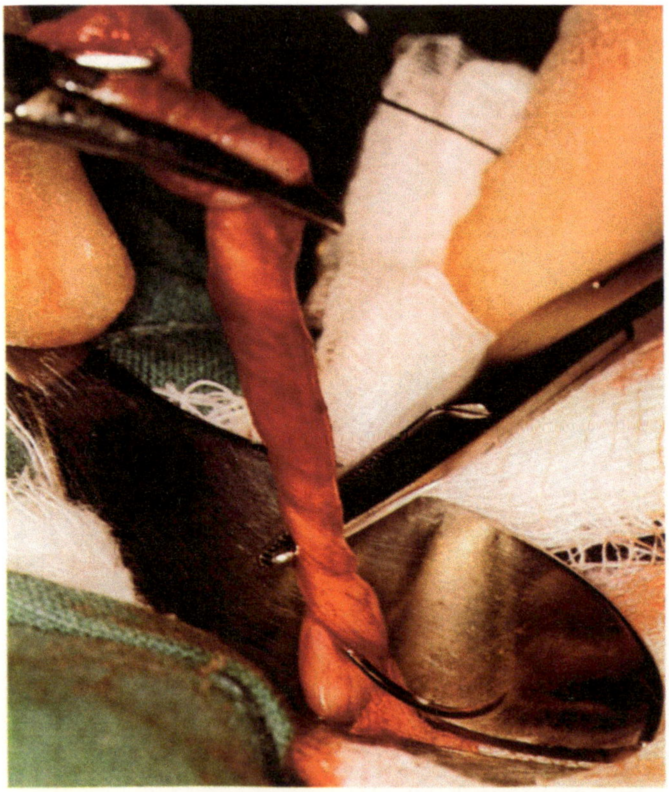

28 A transfixion suture is placed through the hernial sac, avoiding vas and vessels, using 3/0 or 2/0 black silk (size depends on the age of the child and the thickness of the sac).

29

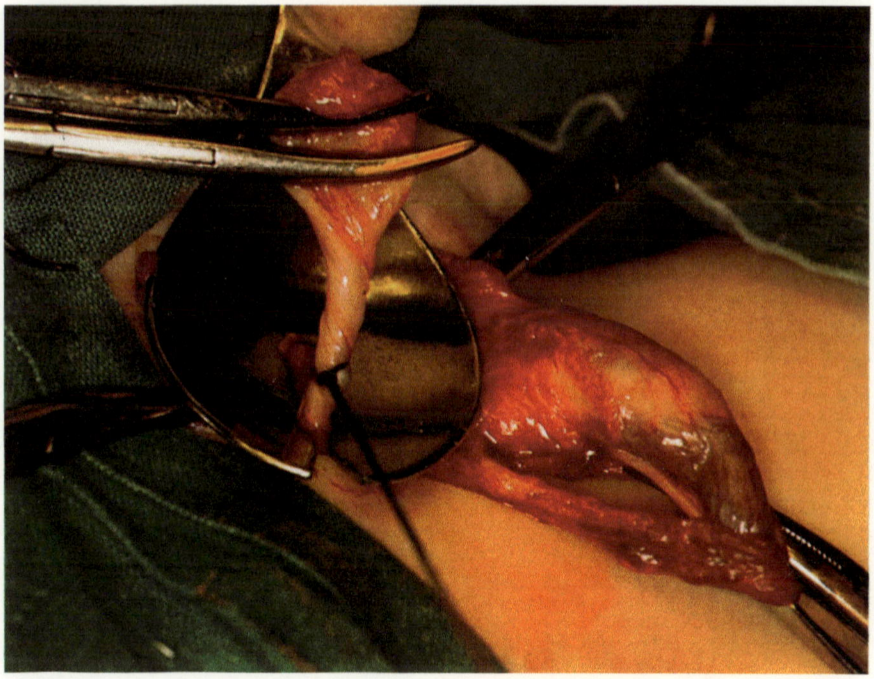

29 Tension of hernial sac. While this suture is being tied the hernial sac is kept on tension so that the suture lies as near the deep inguinal ring as possible.

30

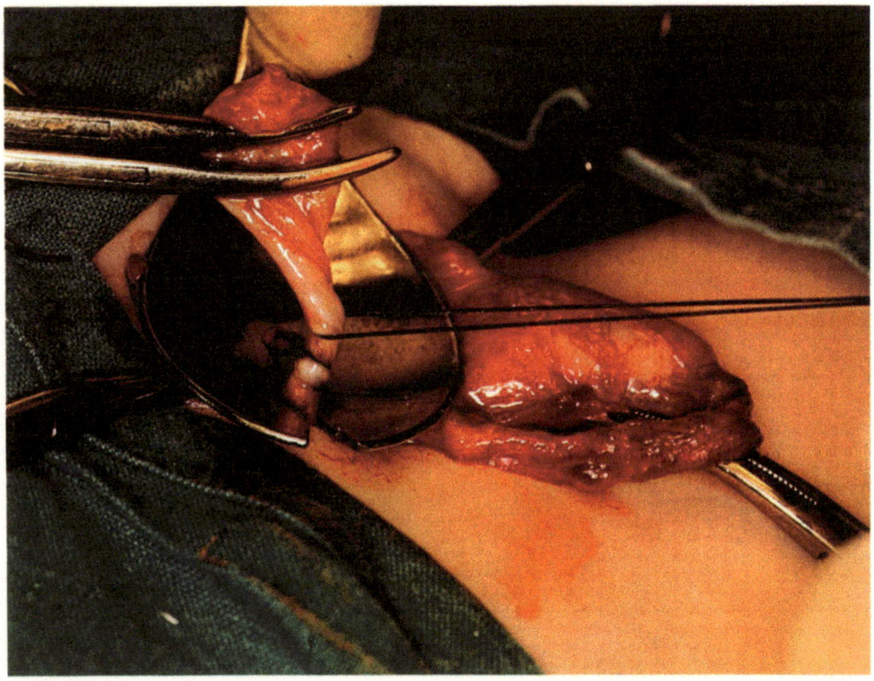

30 A second suture is tied around the hernial sac above the first suture.
This prevents problems should one stitch break or slip.

31

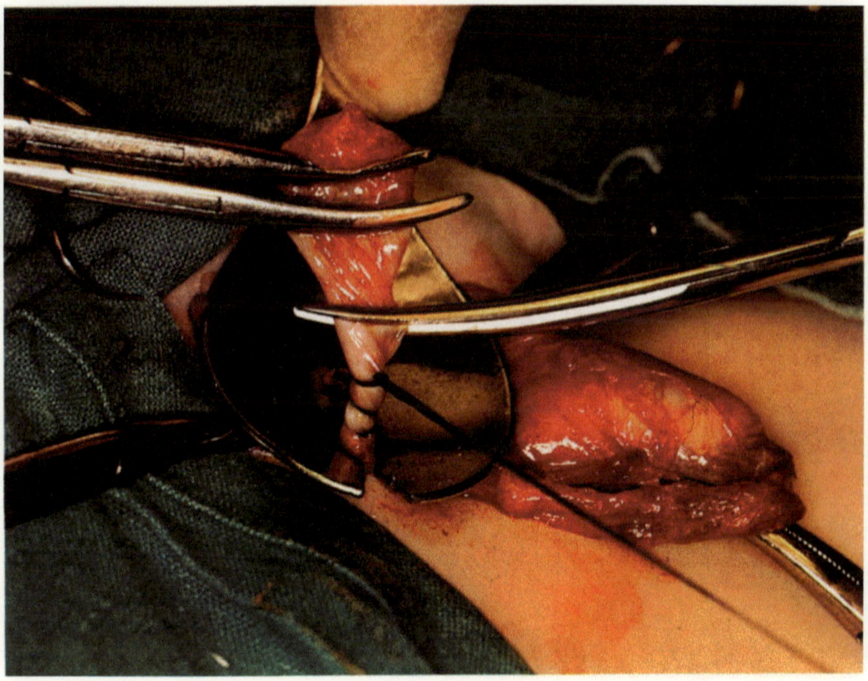

31 While the second stitch is held, the sac is divided distally to the two sutures with the sac under tension.

32

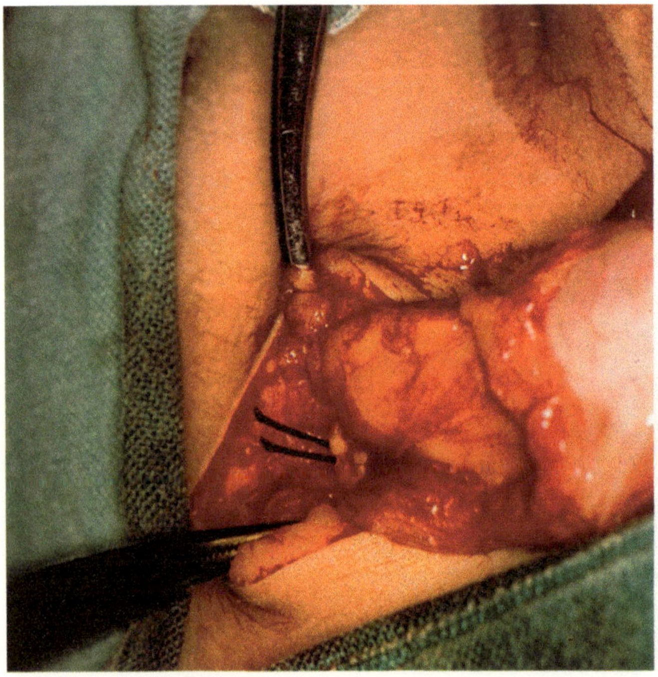

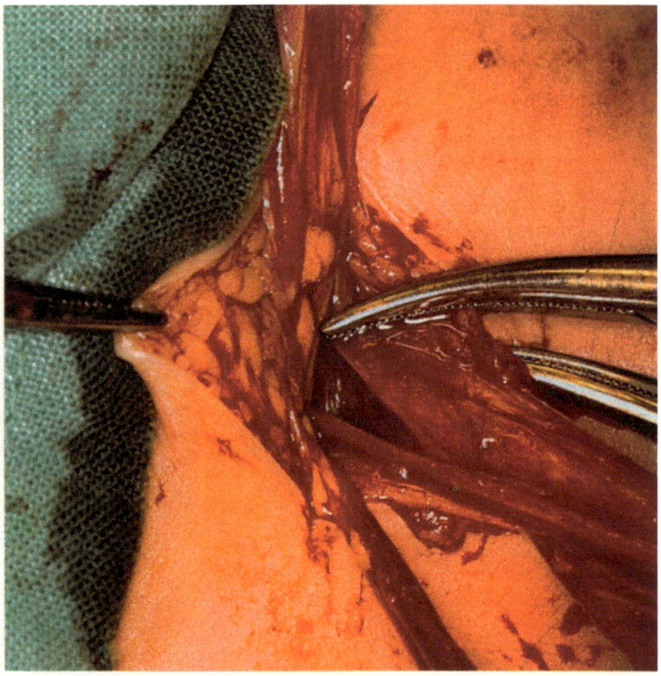

33

32 and 33 If adequate tension has been applied, the stump will disappear into the depths of the wound through the deep inguinal ring once the suture is cut.

34

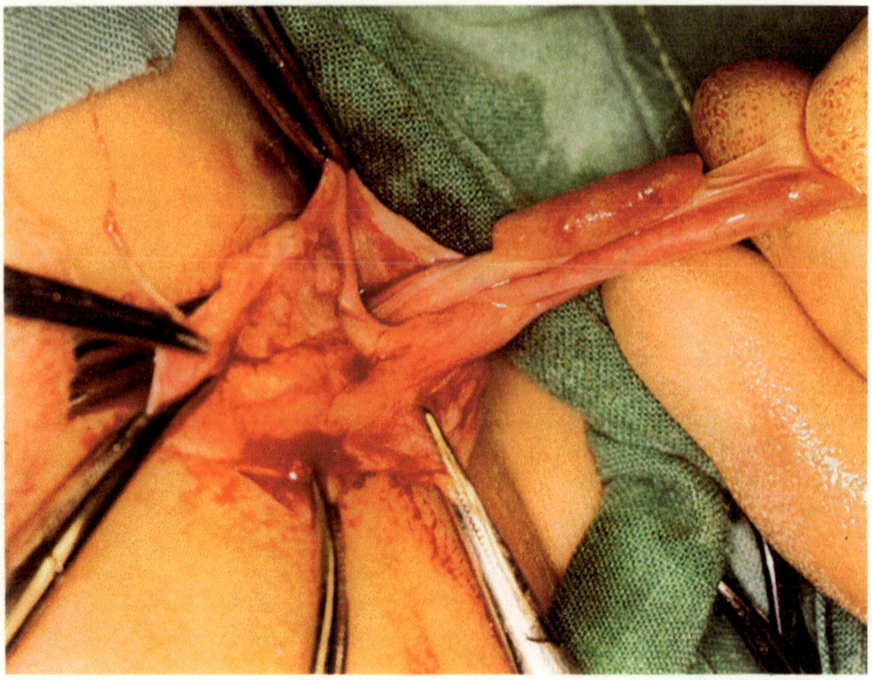

34 Ovary in sac. In female children, when the sac is opened, an ovary may be found in the sac. It should be returned to the abdominal cavity and the hernial sac closed as before.

35

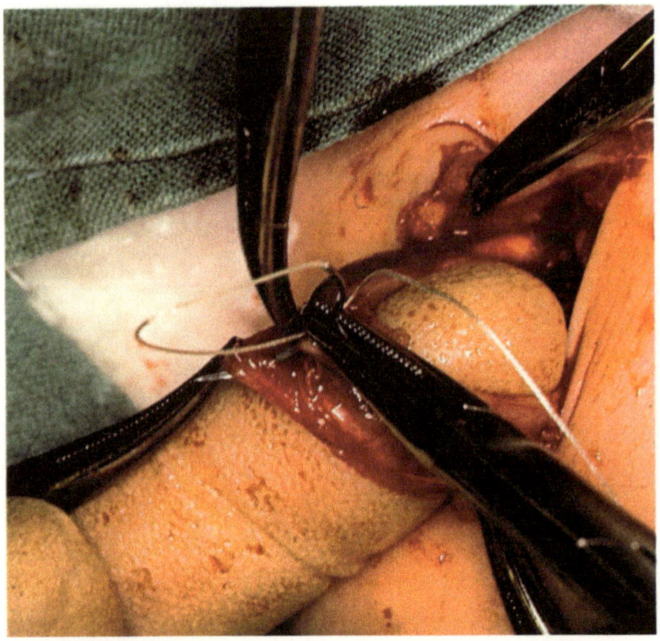

36

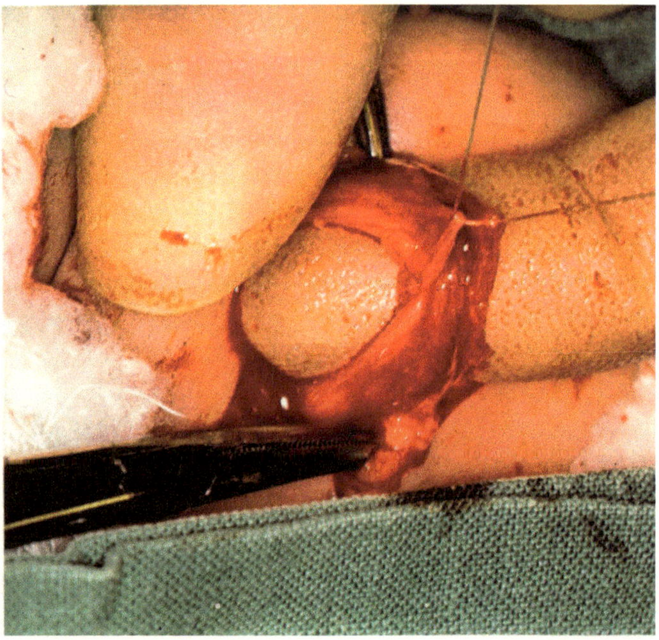

35 The coverings of the cord may be approximated to return the anatomy to as near normal as possible.

36 Only one or two Dexon sutures (3/0) are used. This allows for any collection of blood or oedema to drain.

37 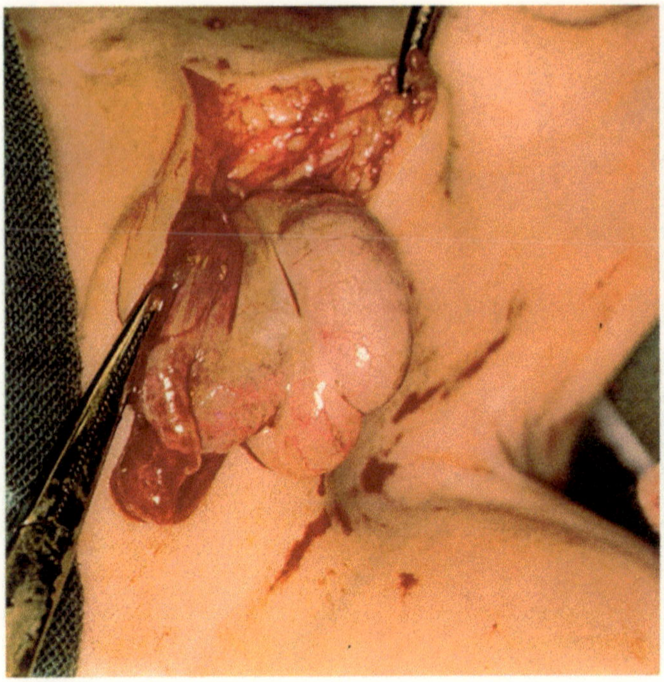

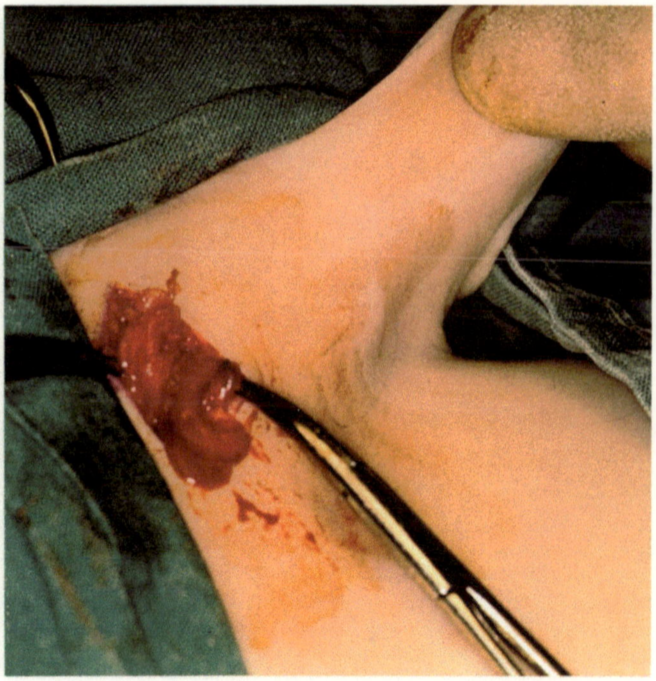 38

37 Undescended testis. As seen in some of the previous photographs, with dissection, the testis may have been brought out of the scrotum. In some children, the testis may be undescended because of the presence of the hernia.

38 By dealing with the hernia the testis is released. It must be replaced in the scrotum to prevent an iatrogenic undescended testis occurring after hernia repair. This is achieved by gentle traction on the scrotum. The vas and vessels must be orientated correctly, so as not to cause torsion and therefore lead to late atrophy of the testis.

39

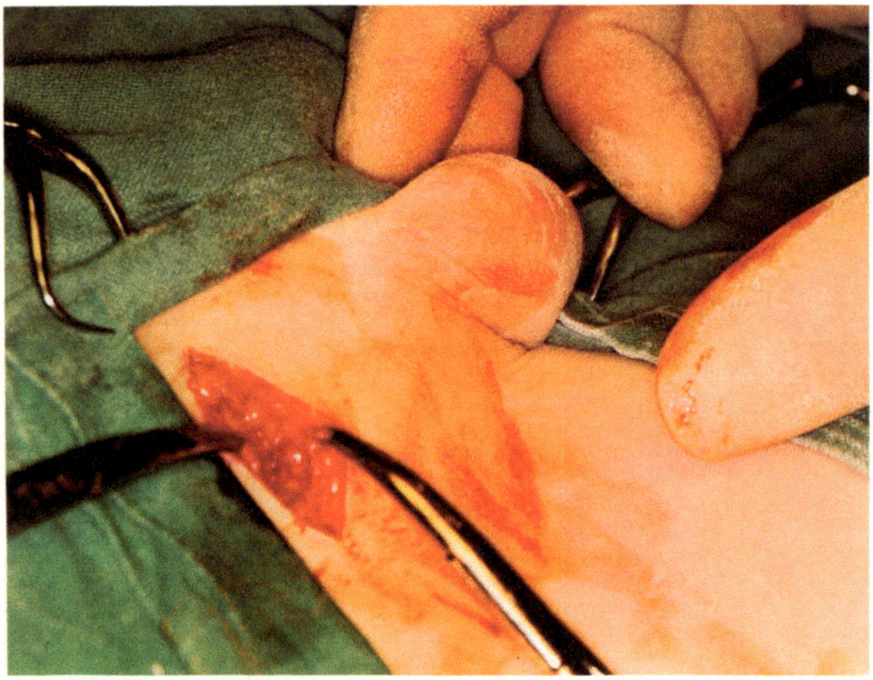

39 The testis is seen in the scrotum. The two clips which were originally put on the wound should still be in place.

40

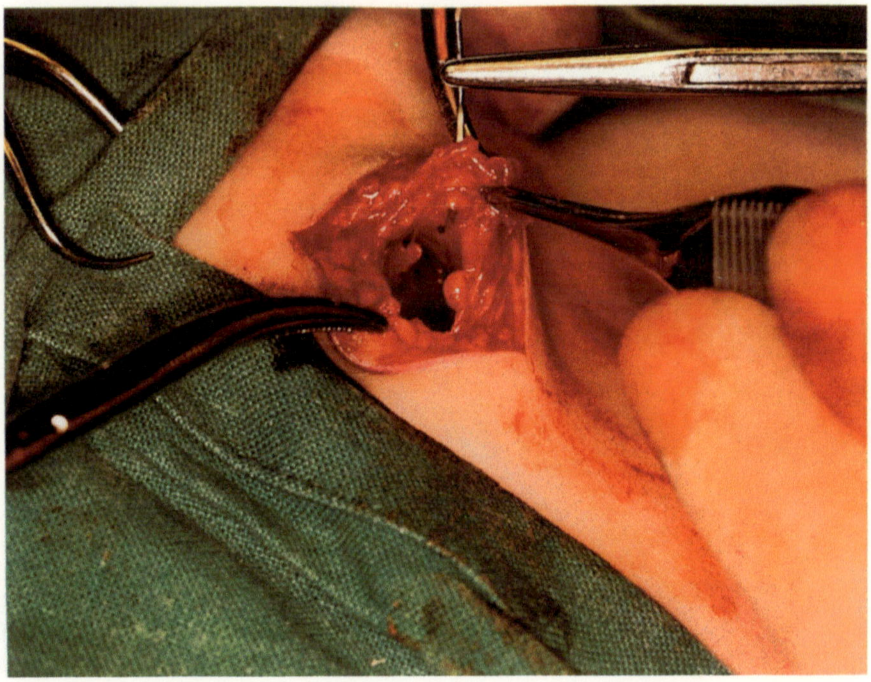

40 Closure of superficial fascia. These clips are held up clear of the deep dissection to allow closure of the superficial fascia. Interrupted subcutaneous sutures of Dexon (3/0) are used to approximate this. Usually only two or three are necessary.

41

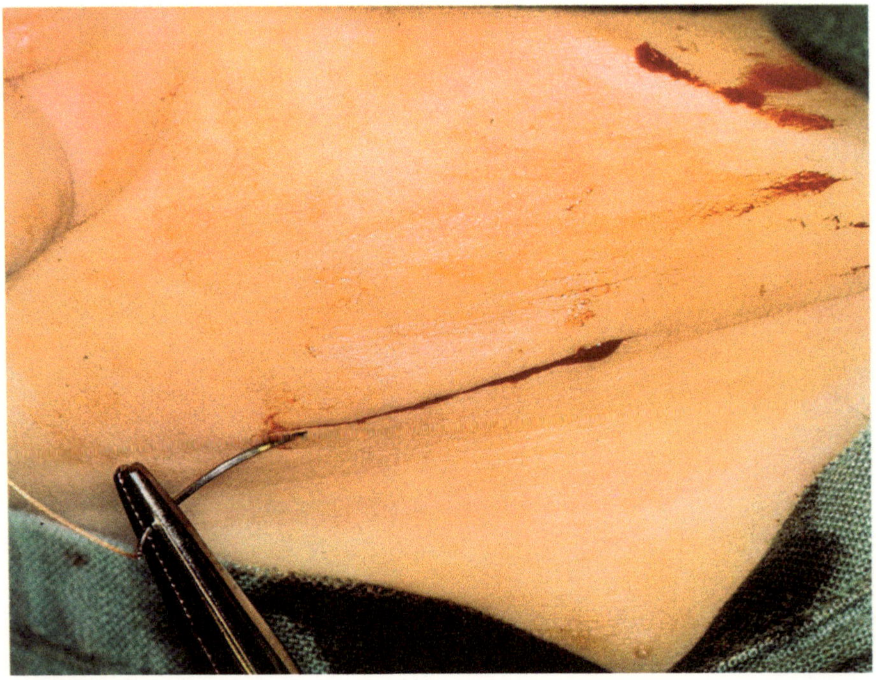

41 If the wound has been placed correctly in a skin crease the two edges will lie together without sutures.

42

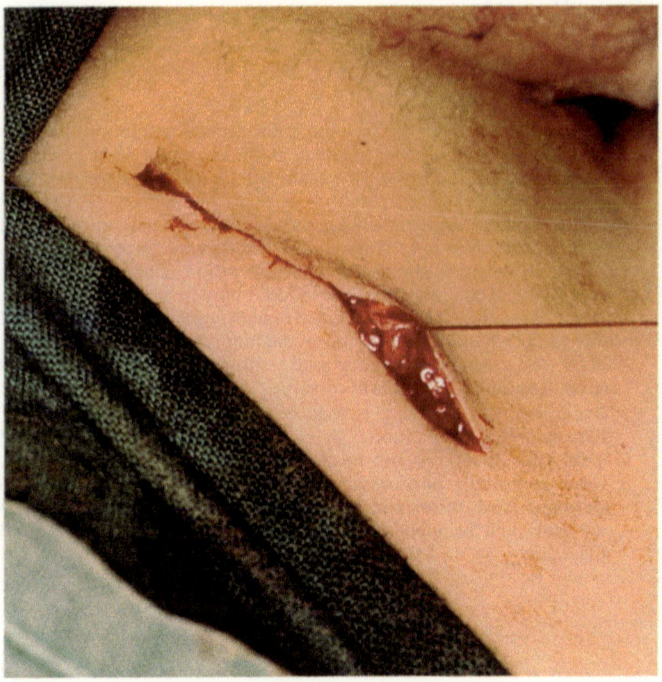

43

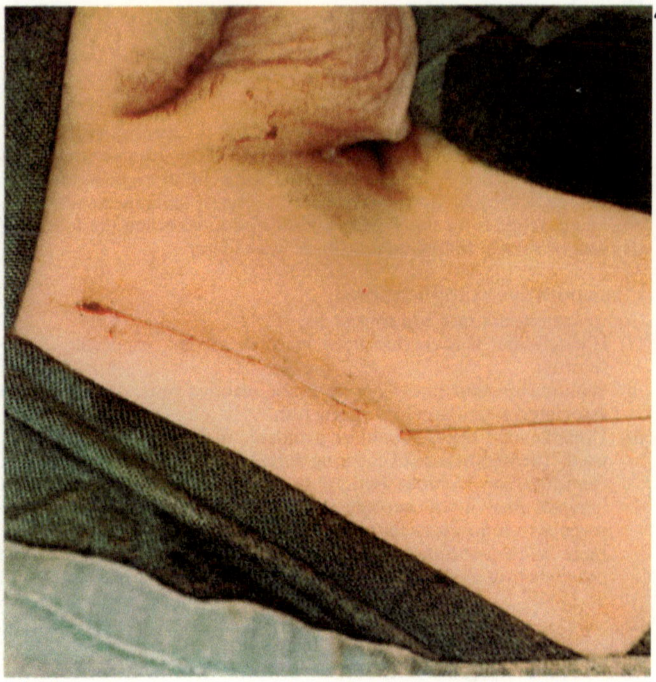

42 and 43 Cosmetic appearance. Subcuticular continuous Dexon suture (3/0) is used for skin closure to give a more cosmetic result. This obviates the necessity for suture removal in very young children. Very occasionally, the use of Dexon may give an indurated scar.

A plastic spray (acrylic resin) may be used with or without a gauze strip as dressing.

Postoperative management and complications

There may be some swelling of the scrotum and the wound, especially if the testis has been brought out of the scrotum. This settles within 24 to 48 hours. The baby or infant can be fed some six to eight hours after surgery, once the patient has recovered completely from the anaesthetic. Normal practice is for the child to be allowed to go home the following day and be seen at follow-up four to six weeks later.

Postoperative complications

Complications are rare and consist of:

i) Haematoma, if there has been much dissection, especially in the scrotum.

ii) Wound infection rarely occurs in the elective case, and is usually associated with a previous nappy rash.

iii) Undescended testes should be avoidable if the proper technique is used. The importance of ensuring the testis is returned to the scrotum cannot be over emphasised. If the testis is left at the superficial inguinal ring, it will become fixed by scar tissue requiring further surgery to return it to the scrotum. In many large hernias in babies, there is an associated undescended testis because the hernial sac prevents proper descent of the testis. In these cases the testis should be placed and fixed in the scrotum at the time of herniotomy.

If the testis has been involved with ischaemia as a result of incarceration of the bowel, the testis will atrophy over the next few years.

iv) If structures are dissected with great care, damage to ovaries, testes, bowel and bladder is unlikely. The risk of damage to cord structures and sac contents is increased if the operation is performed as an emergency. Remember that the bladder may be involved as part of the medial wall of a direct hernia. This can look like peritoneum and only the production of urine gives the hint of the true abnormality. Once the mistake is recognised, suture of the bladder and catheterisation is all that is necessary.

v) The chance of recurrence is reduced by performing elective rather than emergency operations, by careful technique in handling and identifying structures and by avoiding elaborate 'muscle repairs'. These are totally unnecessary in children and lead to damage to spermatic cord, testes and femoral vessels. Recurrence is rare (0.3 per cent) and usually happens only if it has been a complicated dissection.

44

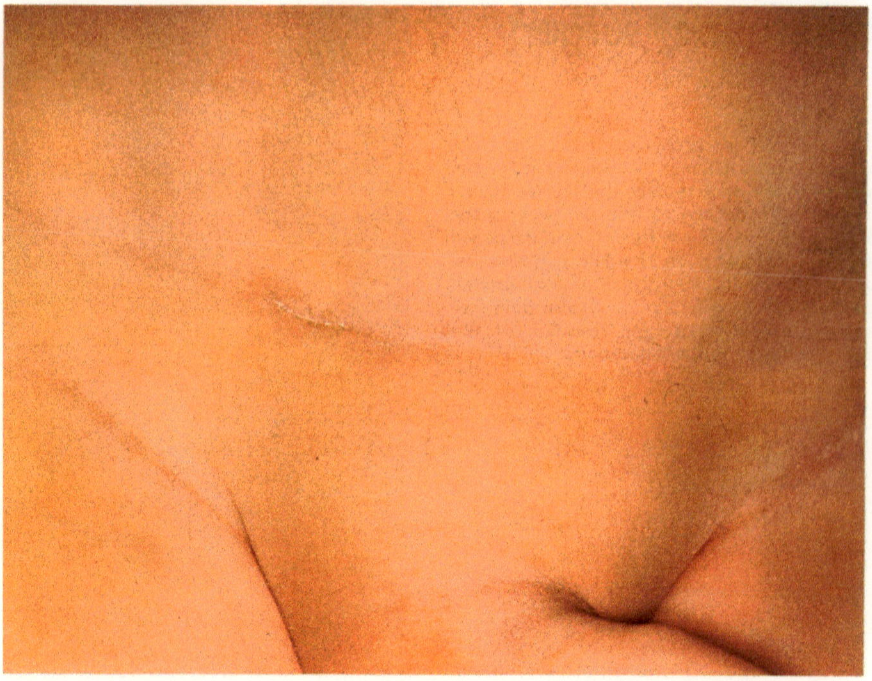

44 Scar placement. A correctly placed scar should be practically invisible some six months later.

Emergency surgery

In the case of the irreducible hernia, the same surgical approach may be possible as in the elective case, but usually the inguinal canal needs to be opened to free the neck of the hernial sac and to allow the return of the bowel to the peritoneal cavity. I would suggest a low incision in the iliac fossa which allows dissection at the external inguinal ring, but also entry into the abdominal cavity for resection of the necrotic bowel, if that is necessary.

45

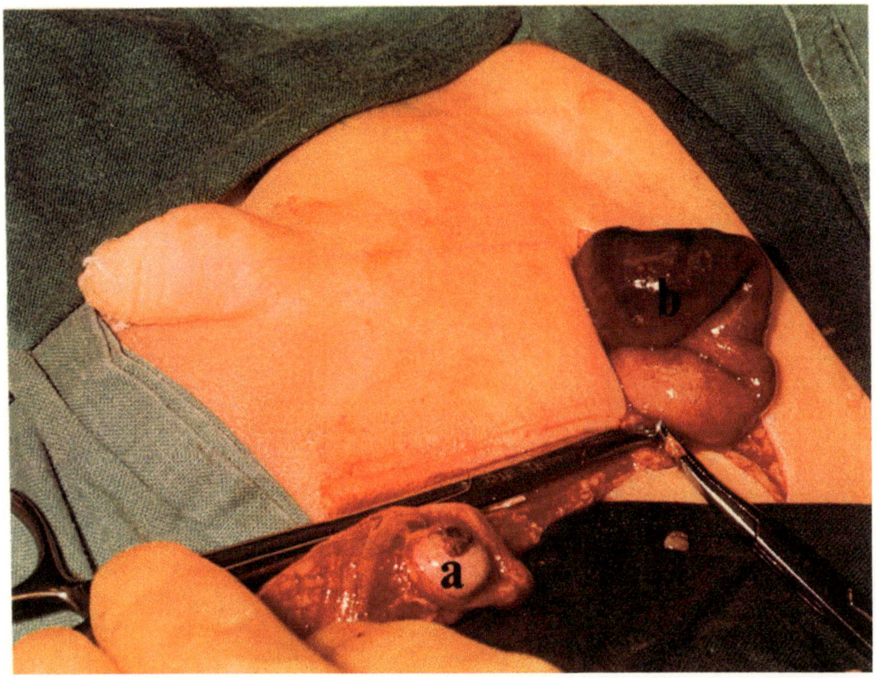

45 Incision in emergency operation. In the emergency operation for an obstructed inguinal hernia, a larger incision is necessary and the testis must be brought out. When the hernial sac is opened, if the bowel is gangrenous, resection must be carried out. A further abdominal incision may be necessary as above – (**a**) the testis at the inguinal incision and (**b**) necrotic bowel at the abdominal incision.

Although it is tempting after resection of necrotic bowel to reanastomose the bowel, in the very young and/or premature baby, the fashioning of stomas may be safer. Closure of the stomas can be carried out within the next three to six weeks, when the child is in a far better condition.

Hydroceles

46

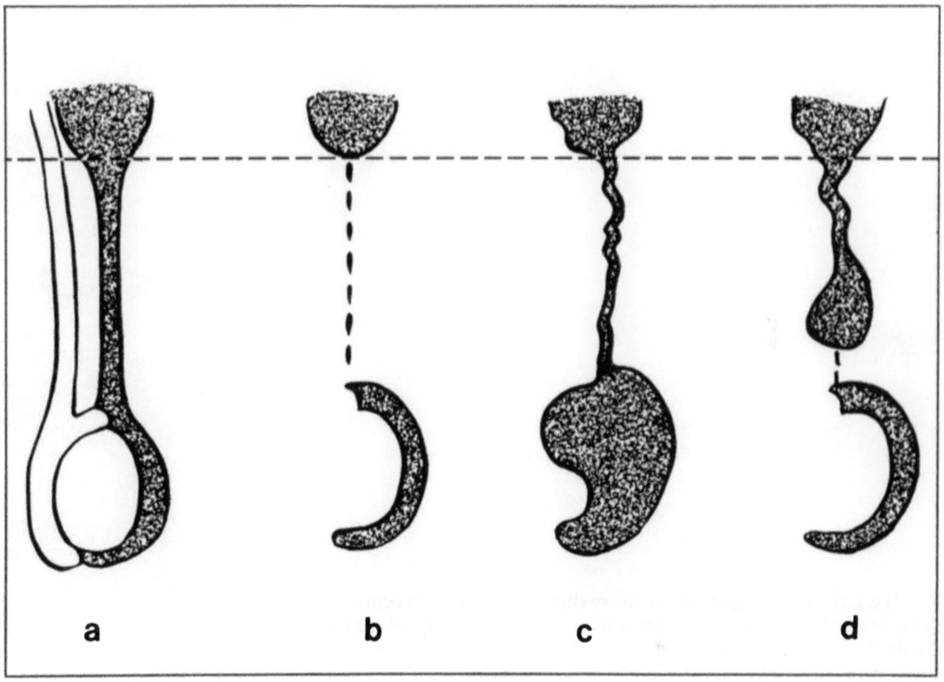

Congenital hydroceles occur because of the persistence of the processus vaginalis. Different types of hydrocele occur depending on the part of the processus remaining.

46 Types of hydroceles.
a) Intact processus vaginalis.
b) Normal anatomy.
c) Hydrocele.
d) Hydrocele of the cord.
As long as no associated inguinal hernia is involved, there is no urgency to treat hydroceles in infants, because most resolve when the processus vaginalis atrophies. It is usually unnecessary to operate before the child reaches two years of age. However, when an acute hydrocele occurs, especially in the infant or child, the possibility that it is masking torsion of the testis must be kept in mind. In all cases, the superficial inguinal ring must be checked thoroughly to exclude an indirect inguinal hernia.

47

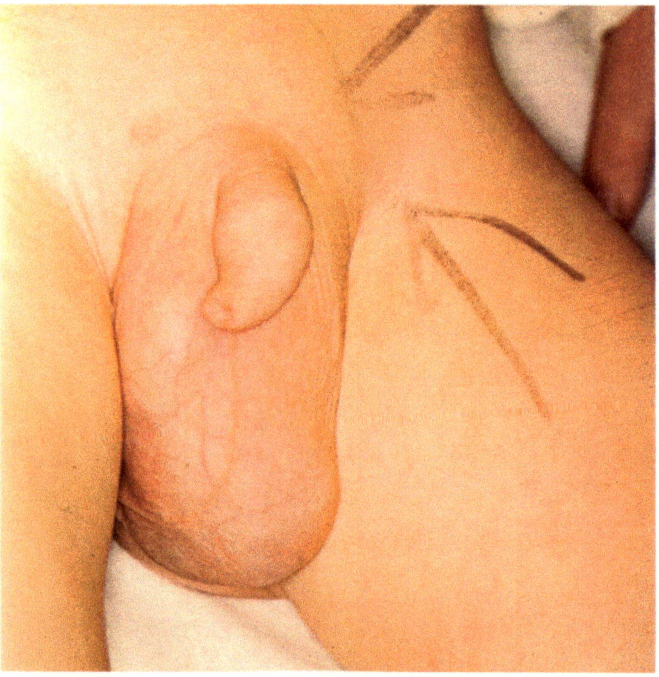

47 It is possible to palpate above the swelling which will not reduce. In the case of a hydrocele of the cord a similar swelling is palpable at the inguinal ring. The arrow indicates the side to be operated on and not the swelling.

48

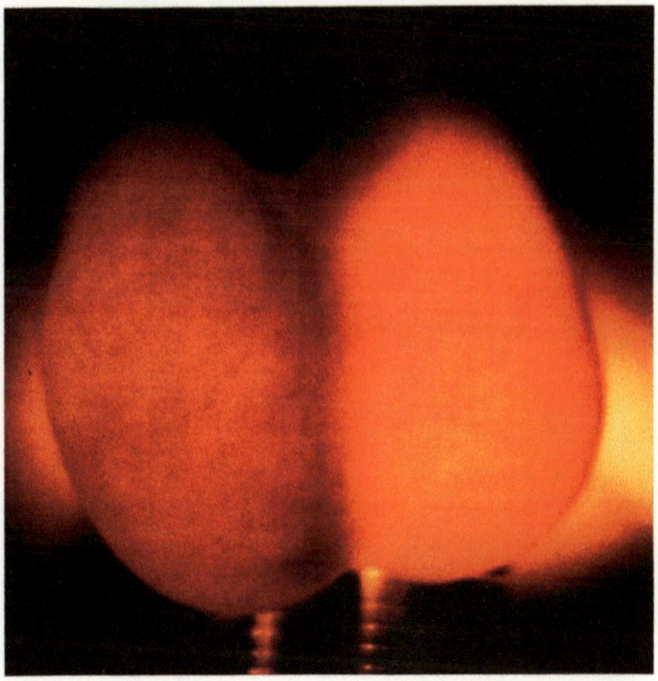

48 The swelling can be transilluminated – in this case in bilateral hydroceles.

Surgery on hydroceles [49]

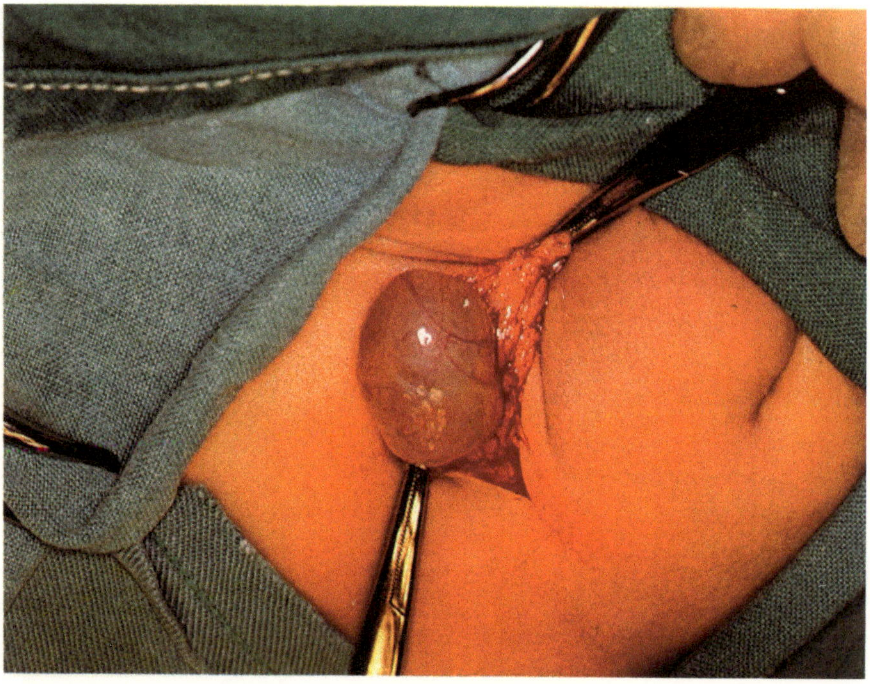

Treatment is by ligation of the proximal part of the processus allowing drainage of the distal portion. The operation for dealing with hydroceles in children is similar to that for baby hernias. The incision is the same, with dissection towards the superficial ring, up to **14**.

49 Hydroceles of the cord may bulge out through the wound even before dissection of the cord is carried out.

50

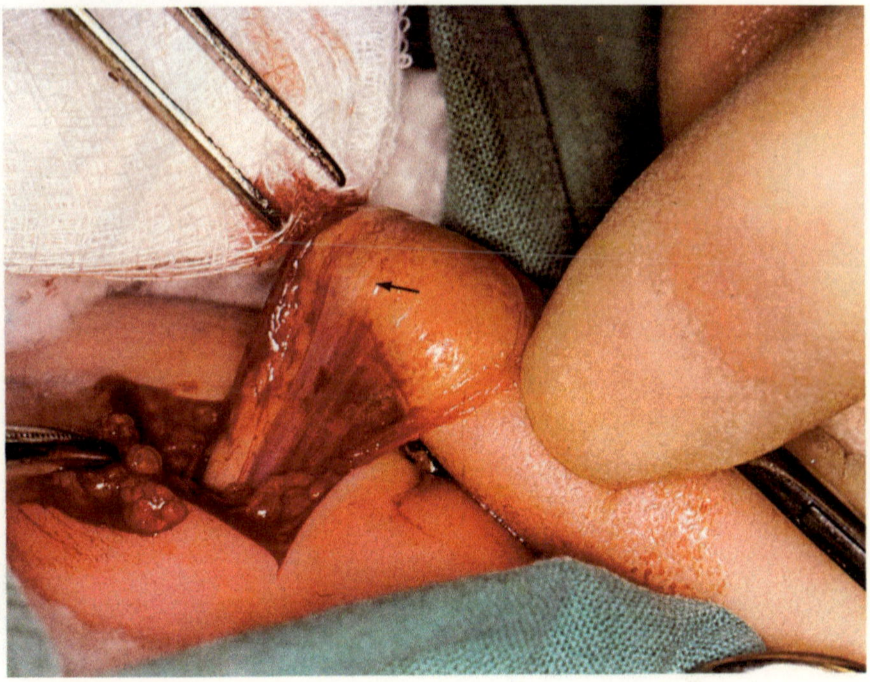

50 However, in the more common scrotal hydrocele the processus (arrowed) can be visualised, when the cord is brought out of the wound and placed over the index finger as before.

51

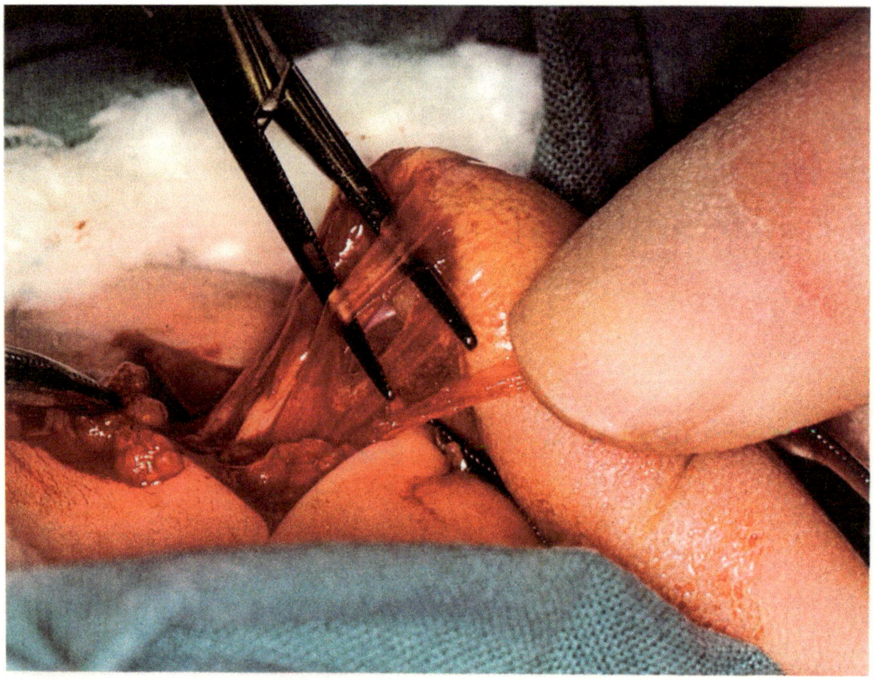

51 After division of the coverings the processus is dissected free from the rest of the tissues in the cord.

52 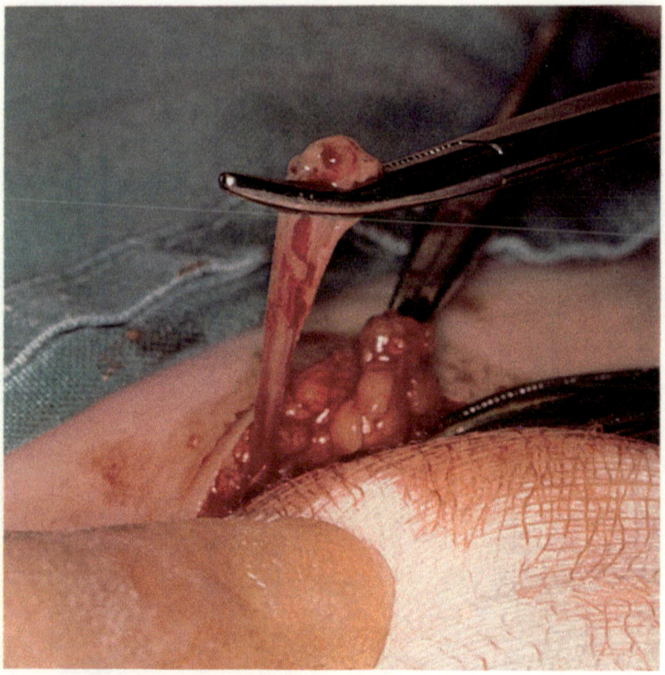 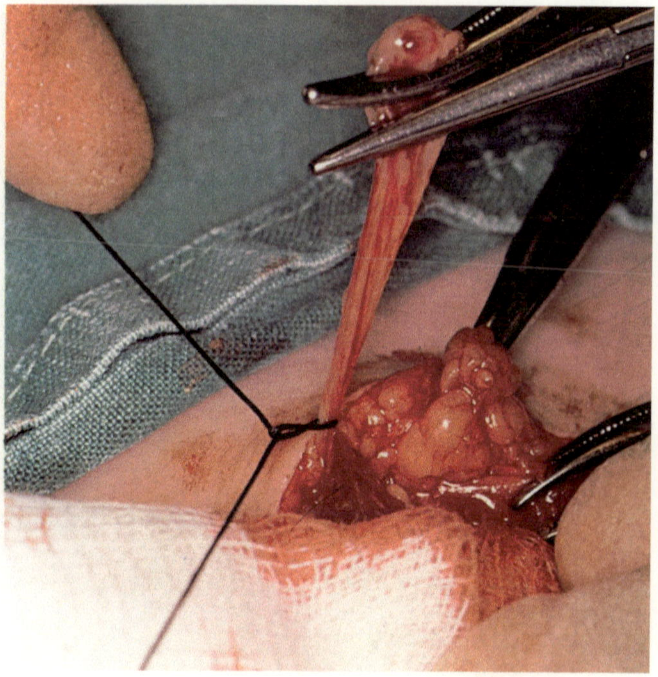 53

52 A clip is placed across the processus which is then divided distally. There is no need for the testis to be brought out into the wound.

53 Two clips are used so that the processus vaginalis can be dissected proximally to the deep inguinal ring. Again under tension, the processus is doubly ligated as near the ring as possible.

54

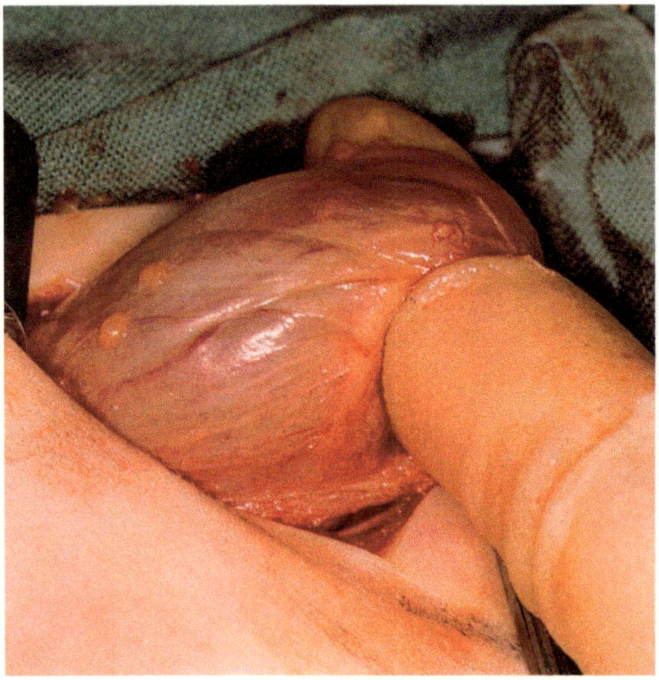

55

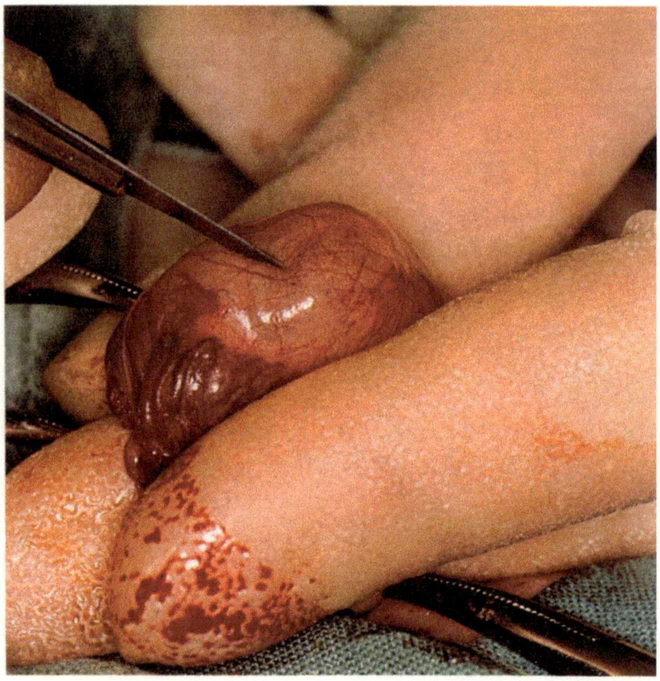

54 After division of the processus the freed distal portion will allow drainage of the fluid. However, some hydroceles may not empty spontaneously. They should be allowed to bulge into the wound.

55 Care being taken to prevent damage to vas or epididymis; the hydrocele is incised to allow drainage. No further surgery is required on the distal portion in children.

56

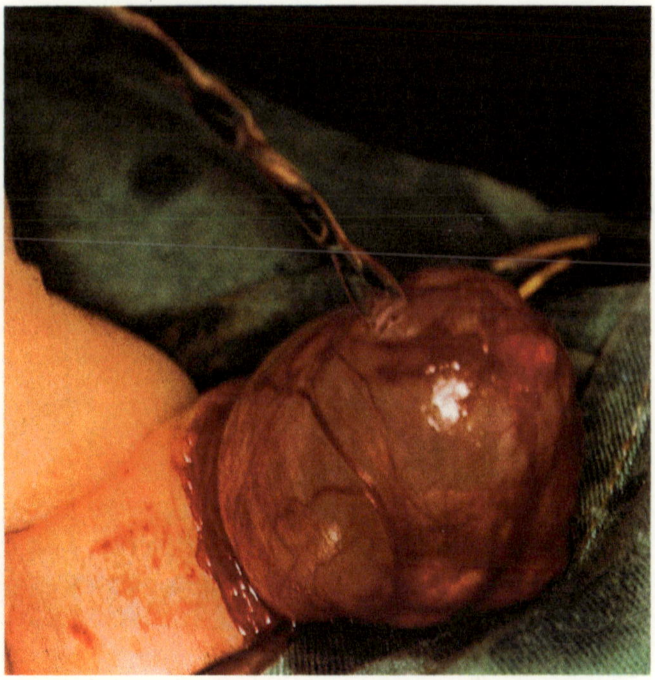

56 Here the clear fluid is draining from a small incision in the tunica vaginalis. The testis is returned to the scrotum and the closure is the same as for closure following surgery for hernias (see **35** onwards).

57

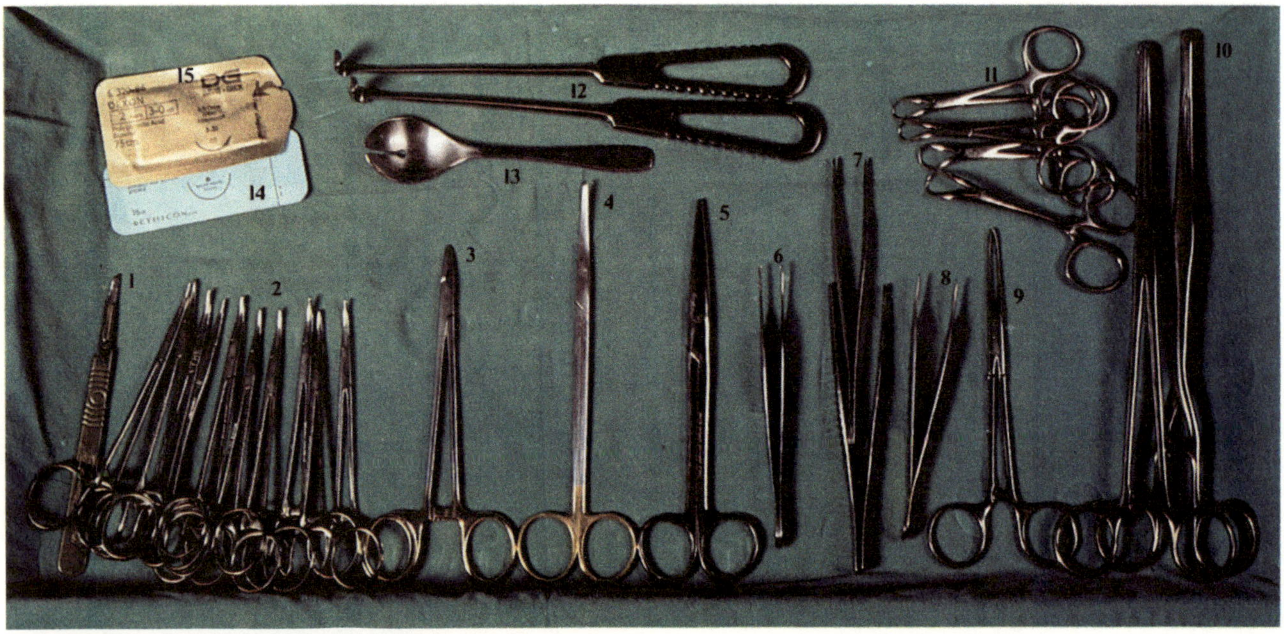

57 Instruments most commonly used in hernia and hydrocele operations.

1 No. 3 Bard Parker handle with No. 15 blade
2 Curved Halstead's mosquito forceps
3 Cryle–Wood needle holder
4 Metzenbaum scissors 7″
5 Suture scissors
6 Adson's toothed dissecting forceps
7 Blunt ended non-toothed dissecting forceps
8 Adson's diamond jaw non-toothed dissecting forceps
9 Allis tissue forceps
10 Rampley's sponge-holding forceps
11 Backhaus towel clips
12 Small Langenbeck retractors
13 Split spoon (Denis Browne)
14 2/0 silk atraumatic suture on round-bodied needle
15 3/0 Dexon on multi-purpose needle

Postoperative course

Postoperative care after hydrocele operation is the same as for a child who has had an inguinal herniotomy.

Complications arising after hydrocele surgery are similar to those mentioned following inguinal herniotomy. Swelling of the scrotum almost always occurs, but this settles within two to three days.

When the processus vaginalis has been left intact by treating the hydrocele either by aspiration or by opening it via the scrotum, the hydrocele will recur. The risk of iatrogenic undescended testis also follows hydrocele surgery.

References

1 Atwell, J., *Paediatric Surgery* (Ed. Nixon, H.H.) (Rob, C. and Smith, R.) 'Operative Surgery', Butterworths, 1978.

2 Jones, Peter G., *Clinical Paediatric Surgery – Diagnosis and Management*, John Wright & Sons, 1970.

3 Holder, T.M. and Ashcraft, K.W., *Pediatric Surgery*, W.B. Saunders, 1980.

4 Nixon, H.H., *Surgical Conditions in Paediatrics*, Butterworths, 1978.

Index

Numbers in medium indicate page numbers; those in **bold** indicate caption and figure numbers.